THE ULTIMATE PATH TO SUCCESS

D1401778

THE ULTIMATE PAth TO SUCCESS

A Road Map for Physician Assistant School Applicants

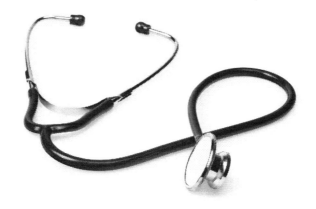

Andrew J. Rodican, PA-C

andrewrodican.com

ISBN-10: 1519705778

ISBN-13: 9781519705778

Library of Congress Control Number: 2015920364

Createspace Independent Publishing Platform, North Charleston, SC

Book design and production by Greg Johnson/Textbook Perfect

Cover images © megaflopp/Shutterstock; ducu59us/Shutterstock. Andrew Rodican image supplied by the author.

Printed in the United States of America

10 9 8 7 6 5 4 3 2 1

This book is dedicated to my family . . .

*My beautiful wife Allison, whom I love with all my heart
and who supports me in good times and bad.*

*My son Eddie, who is currently on his own path to becoming a PA
and makes me proud to be his father;
and his wife Lizzie, the best daughter-in-law a father could ask for.*

*My daughter Nicole, who has worked extremely hard
to achieve all of her goals in life
and is a power of example in her profession.*

*My son Andrew, who makes me smile every day and has more energy
than should be allowed by law.*

*My little sweetheart Natalie, who is as stubborn as her older sister,
and has the eyes to melt my heart.*

*And finally, my gorgeous granddaughter Lyla,
who lights up my heart with pride and joy.*

I am truly blessed!

Contents

ABOUT THE AUTHOR

Andrew J. Rodican, PA-C, is a 1994 graduate of the Yale University School of Medicine Physician Associate Program. Rodican served on the admission's committee at Yale for three years, both as a student and graduate member. He has been writing books and coaching PA school applicants to success since 1996. Andrew has a strong passion for the PA profession and for helping those who desire to pursue this career path.

Andrew published his first book, *The Ultimate Guide to Getting into Physician Assistant School*, in 1996. This book was the first of its kind and is now in its third edition. This book is the gold standard for those who want to pursue a career as a physician assistant. He went on to publish two more books, *How to "Ace" the Physician Assistant School Interview* and *Essays That Will Get You into Physician Assistant School*.

Rodican is also a seasoned and passionate PA-school applicant coach, having helped thousands of PA-school applicants achieve acceptance to programs all over the country. He offers counseling sessions, essay review and editing services, mock interviews, and an informative website exclusively designed for you, the PA-school applicant. You can find Andrew's website at www.andrewrodican.com.

Andrew is also an accomplished clinician, having served as a PA in many specialty areas including cardiothoracic surgery, occupational medicine, cardiology, and bariatric medicine. Andrew was the founder of Medical Weight Loss Centers in East Haven, Connecticut, and owned one of the prominent single weight-loss clinics in the United States for eight years. In 2009, Andrew was one of only four midlevel clinicians to pass the bariatric medicine board-certification examination through the American Board of Bariatric Medicine.

Andrew currently works in family practice and internal medicine and continues to see bariatric patients as part of his duties.

Preface

Each time I find myself writing another book, I'm fortunate to keep emphasizing that the physician assistant (PA) profession is currently one of the top career fields in the country and is projected to grow significantly over the next several years. That's the good news!

The bad news is that competition for getting accepted to a PA program is fierce. Many applicants become frustrated with the application process and don't know where to turn for answers. They have questions like,

- ▸ What is the best type of medical experience to obtain?
- ▸ Is my GPA high enough?
- ▸ How do I find PAs to shadow?
- ▸ How many PAs should I shadow?
- ▸ How do I write a great essay?
- ▸ What questions will I be asked at my interview?

The list can go on and on. Many applicants will seek out the advice of PA friends or PA forums on the Internet. This is an OK strategy, but you will be getting biased advice from PAs who only know how the process works at the school they attended. But what if one school asks all traditional interview questions and another asks all behavioral questions? Some schools use multiple mini-interviews (MMI's) during the interview. Unless your sources are familiar with all of the information from every school, your chances are less than average.

My unique background and years of experience allow me to coach applicants from a global perspective rather than a narrow one. You don't have to go it alone. This workbook will prepare you for the entire application process and clarify all of your questions and concerns.

Congratulations on choosing the best profession in the world.

Introduction

Since 1996, I've had the priviledge of coaching thousands of physician assistant school applicants achieve their dream of becoming physician assistant students. Through my books and personal coaching services, I find that I benefit as much from helping applicants as the applicants benefit from my products and services. Each time I work with PA school applicants via coaching sessions, mock-interview sessions, and reading and editing their essays, I learn more and more about their needs. The common threads tying these applicants together include a strong passion for becoming a PA and the need for a road map to help them achieve success. The PA profession and PA programs are constantly in flux. The physician assistant school application process can be overwhelming at times. *The Ultimate PAth to Success* will help you learn everything about the application process and will provide you with the laser-like focus necessary to achieve your dream of becoming a certified physician assistant (PA-C).

This book is a workbook meant to supplement my other books and individual coaching sessions. This material includes powerful techniques and exercises that will help you maximize your chances for success when applying to PA school. However, you must thoroughly read and assimilate this information in order for it to work. Mark this book up, and make it yours. Accomplish all of the exercises, and you will be amazed before you are halfway through.

Most of the information included in this workbook does not come from my previous books; it is meant to be a companion guide. This is truly bonus material. I encourage you to grasp the concepts and principles in this material rather than trying to memorize the information verbatim. This workbook contains key information on every aspect of the application process.

I find the essay and interview are the most important parts of the PA school application process. In fact, these two components are the only ones you have any control over. In this workbook, I provide you with detailed information, tips, and exercises on how to write a killer essay. I've spent a great deal of time trying to give you examples of what should be included in a powerful and persuasive essay, along with sample essays that worked for others. I don't expect you to relate directly to each essay; rather, I want you to relate to the principles. The essay is a very personal statement and may be the most important piece of medical writing you will accomplish in your entire medical career. Only you can do an effective job of creating the emotional impact required to connect with the reader.

As far as the interview section is concerned, I not only want you to pay attention to the questions and answers you're most likely to be asked at your interview, I want you to understand and assimilate the different types of interview questions that you are most likely to be asked. The interview chapter covers traditional questions, behavioral questions, situational questions, ethical questions, illegal questions, multiple mini interview (MMI) questions, and "if you were a color/animal/tree/fruit, what would it be" questions. You can find an entire list of each format; including answers to every question you might be asked, in my book titled *How to "Ace" the Physician Assistant School Interview*.

Finally, an understanding of the PA profession is a key selection factor. The first several pages of this focus pack will educate you on current issues, including message points that were published by the American Academy of Physician Assistants (AAPA) to be used by PAs during National PA Week in 2010. These message points represent issues the AAPA wants to put out to the media about our profession. These key points will be valuable to know for interviews and for your general knowledge of current issues in the profession.

I also strongly suggest that you join the American Academy of Physician Assistants as an affiliate member and your state, or constituent, chapter of the AAPA. For the modest investment you make to join these organizations, you will receive a constant stream of current information relative to the PA profession. This information will help you through the entire application process. OK, buckle up, get a pencil ready, and let's start the journey on your PAth to success.

Andrew J. Rodican, PA-C
March 2016

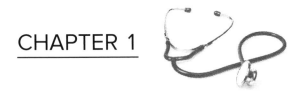

CHAPTER 1

History of the PA Profession

In 1965 Dr. Eugene Stead of the Duke University Medical Center in North Carolina started the first PA program. He is considered the pioneer of the PA profession. The profession got its start because of a shortage and disproportionate distribution of primary-care physicians at the time. The first program was comprised of former navy corpsmen who served in Vietnam and already had considerable clinical experience. These former corpsmen had no avenue for transferring their skills to the civilian world. Dr. Stead trained these corpsmen in a way comparable to the fast-track programs physicians completed during World War II. The profession grew from these first few veterans to over eighty thousand practicing PAs in 2015–2016.

WHAT IS A PHYSICIAN ASSISTANT?

By definition, PAs are "dependent" health care professionals who must always work under the supervision of a licensed physician. Rather than follow their physician colleagues around like puppies, most PAs work autonomously and, typically, collaboratively with their MD supervisors. PAs are broadly trained and perform a variety of duties, depending on the specialty, practice setting, supervising physician, and scope of practice. In general, PAs take a comprehensive medical history and perform physical examinations, formulate diagnoses and treatment plans, order and interpret diagnostic tests, assist in surgery, prescribe medications, counsel patients and family members, perform minor surgical procedures, and consult with their supervising physicians on a regular basis.

PAs are found in almost every area and specialty of medical and surgical practice. About half of all PAs work in primary care (family practice, obstetrics and gynecology, pediatrics, and internal medicine). Another 20 percent of PAs work in the various surgical specialties, and the remainder of PAs works in a host of other specialty and subspecialty arenas. Some PAs actually own their own practices and hire supervising physicians to work as their medical directors.

HOW ARE PAs TRAINED?

Most PA programs are approximately two years in length. Students are trained in the medical model, similar to most medical school programs. In fact, the didactic phase of a PA program is often equated to the first three years of medical school. Many PA students share certain classes with medical students at those programs affiliated with a medical school. The main difference between physician training and physician assistant training is the number of years physicians are required to spend in residencies after the didactic phase is completed.

The first year of PA school is typically dedicated to the classroom and clinical practicum sessions. PA students can expect to take courses in clinical laboratory sciences, electrocardiography, emergency medicine and trauma, interviewing techniques, medicine and surgery, microbiology and infectious disease, pharmacology, physical examination, physiology and biochemistry, psychodynamics of human behavior, anatomy, diagnostic imaging, epidemiology and public health, ethics, human sexuality, and pathology.

The second year of PA school is geared toward clinical rotations. Most programs have mandatory rotations in emergency medicine, family/general medicine, general surgery, internal medicine, obstetrics and gynecology, pediatrics, and psychiatry. In addition, students can typically choose from a number of elective rotations.

Upon graduating from an accredited PA program, students are eligible to sit for the Physician Assistant National Certifying Examination (PANCE), which is given by the National Commission on Certification of Physician Assistants (NCCPA) in conjunction with the National Board of Medical Examiners. Students are eligible for state licensure after passing the PANCE. PAs must acquire one hundred hours of continuing medical education (CME) every two years and pass the Physician Assistant National Recertification Examination every ten years. The recertification process is currently being reevaluated and will likely change soon.

Message Points

The following message points were included in a tool kit from the 2010 American Academy of Physician Assistants for PA Week. The message was "Celebrating PAs Who Transform Health Care."

> ▸ There are more than eighty thousand [in 2010] PAs providing care all across America. PAs are medical professionals licensed to examine, test, and treat patients with the supervision of a physician as part of the health care team.

- Resident hours may be reduced again this year. PAs are a critical element to maintain the continuity of patient care during and after this transition.

- PAs provide high-quality patient care and maintain continuity of care that is an essential component of the new primary-care/medical-home model of care.

- PAs practice in general-practice settings as well as in specialty settings, such as emergency medicine and oncology. The federal government is the largest employer of PAs.

- Accredited PA programs in universities and academic health centers produce close to six thousand graduates a year. They are entering the medical workforce faster than physicians and already play a role in off-setting the physician shortage.

- The PA profession extends the reach of medicine and the promise of health to the most remote and in-need communities. Without PAs, health care providers in hospitals, private practice, nursing homes, correctional institutions, and other health care settings would be overrun.

- Now that the health care reform bill has passed, more people will be seeking medical care. PAs are an integral part of addressing the new demands for care, especially in primary care and family practices.

- Funding for PA educational programs is currently deficient; Congress must support expansion of PA programs as they develop strategies for addressing health care workforce challenges.

- With the right policies in place, today's PA workforce is uniquely qualified to step in and extend care—immediately—to those who need it. The Federal Employee Compensation Act (www.dm.usda.gov/shmd/comques.htm) needs to be updated to allow PAs to diagnose and treat federal employees who are injured on the job.

- The federal Medicare statute must be amended to allow PAs to order home health and hospice care, as well as to provide hospice care for Medicare beneficiaries.

- In Iraq, a typical Army PA serves as the primary health care provider for about 400 to 750 soldiers. When a wounded soldier returns home, military PAs are on the front lines as key members of the transitional care team, providing critical assessments and determining treatment plans.

The following exercise is meant to reinforce your knowledge of the PA profession and its history:

Exercise: About the PA Profession

Fill in the blanks:

1. The PA profession is a _____ profession.

2. PAs must always work under a _____ license.

3. PAs can work in _____ area of medicine/surgery.

4. Most PAs work _____ and typically, _____ with their MD supervisors.

5. The PA profession began in _____.

6. The founder of the PA profession is Dr. _____.

7. The first PA program began at _____ University.

8. There are over _____ practicing PAs today.

9. PAs are trained in the _____ model similar to most medical schools.

10. The first year of the PA program is dedicated to _____

    and _____ sessions.

11. The second year is geared toward _____.

12. Upon graduation from an _____ PA program, the student

    is eligible to sit for the _____, which is

    given by the _____.

TOP TEN PA PROGRAMS IN THE UNITED STATES

At the time of this writing (2015–2016), the number of PAs working in the United States is expected to grow 39 percent by 2018 (according to the Bureau of Labor Statistics.) This growth trend is expected to continue well into the future. Physician assistant school applicants should strive to get into an established PA program (versus a provisionally accredited program); these programs typically have the best first-time success rates on the national boards (PANCE). If you complete a PA program but can't pass the boards, you can't work!

US News & World Report's Top Ten Physician Assistant Programs in the Country as of 2015

1. Duke University
2. University of Iowa
3. Emory University
4. George Washington University
5. Oregon Health & Sciences University
6. Quinnipiac University
7. University of Colorado
8. University of Utah
9. University of Nebraska Medical Center
10. Wake Forest University

Once you become a certified physician assistant (PA-C), you can look forward to a rewarding career field with excellent growth potential and a great salary.

Physician Assistant Career Growth

Year	Number of PAs
1967	4
1975	3,700
2000	40,000
2010	80,000
2018	110,400 (projected)

Salaries for physician assistants are excellent and continue to grow.

Physician Assistant Salary Profile (2015)

10%	$ 80,262
25%	$ 87,477
Median	**$ 95,402**
75%	$104,847
90%	$113,446
95%	$125,000+

Most new graduate PAs start out at the lower to median range of the salary spectrum. However, depending on physician assistant specialty areas of practice, it's possible to start out in the top 75th percentile. If you decide to become a partner or sole owner of a medical practice, your earnings potential is unlimited.

SUMMARY

The physician assistant profession is one of the hottest career fields in medicine right now and is projected to continue growing well into the future. However, competition for getting accepted into PA school remains fierce. Applicants must demonstrate a strong passion for this profession and the motivation to do what is necessary to become a top prospect. To be most competitive, applicants must have a strong knowledge base of the profession. This book will provide you with that knowledge.

While reading this book, begin thinking about how you personally meet or exceed the following eleven scoring criteria that the admissions committees use to evaluate you as a candidate:

1. Understanding of the PA profession
2. Academic ability and test scores
3. Maturity
4. Passion for the PA profession
5. Ability to handle stress
6. Likeliness to be a good fit for the program
7. Knowledge of the programs you apply to
8. Credibility
9. Trust
10. Likeability
11. Health care experience

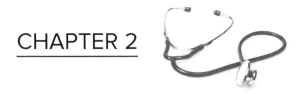

CHAPTER 2

Why Do You Want to Become a Physician Assistant?

I suggest that every applicant applying to PA school be able to answer the question, "Why do you want to be a physician assistant?" in no more than three to four hundred words. The answer goes to the heart of the first element of scoring criteria, "Understanding of the PA profession," listed at the end of the previous chapter. In my experience as an admissions committee member at Yale's PA program from 1994–1996 and coaching thousands of PA school applicants since 1997, I've found most candidates struggle with this key question. If you cannot answer this simple question, then you are likely to struggle with your essay and your interview (if you make it that far).

The following is a typical response that many applicants provide to this question:

I've always been fascinated [very clichéd, by the way] *by medicine. I want to be able to help people and make a difference in their lives. I enjoy working on a team, and I have a strong desire to utilize my science background in a positive way. I have had the opportunity to go on several missions where we helped hundreds of people in poor countries establish medical clinics and housing facilities. I care deeply about these people, and I want to be able to do more for them in a higher capacity.*

I have had the opportunity to shadow three PAs, and I find that they spend a lot more time with patients than their physician counterparts. I see myself working in an orthopedic practice someday. I feel that patients come to an orthopedic surgeon with pain and broken body parts. The orthopedic surgeon takes these patients into the operating room, and they come out "fixed." It's an amazing and fascinating process where you get to see the results of your work instantly, unlike working in an emergency room where you may never see your patients again once they are transferred to another floor or leave the ER to go home.

I have a strong science background with a high GPA and two thousand hours of clinical experience. I think I am a good fit for this profession.

Does this answer the question being asked: Why do you want to become a physician assistant? No, it does not answer the question. One could ask this applicant who is "fascinated" by medicine, why not become a nurse, a nurse practitioner, a paramedic, or a physician? If you want to help people, why not become a firefighter, a police officer, or a customer-service representative in a department store? Why not use your science background to be a researcher or a scientist? If you want to help people in poor, underserved countries, why not become a carpenter and go back to build houses and clinics?

One could also ask, How do you know that you want to work in an orthopedic practice? Have you worked in orthopedics before? Do you know that the mission of most PA programs is to have their graduates work in family practice or underserved areas?

Having a strong science background, a high GPA, and many hours of clinical experience is great—but it still doesn't answer the question!

Here is how I would answer the question:

Having worked as a medical assistant for the past few years, I find that I enjoy working with patients and playing a small role in preparing them for their office visit. However, I now find that I have a strong desire to work in an enhanced role and be able to diagnose and treat these patients. I've done my research on several professions, and I've found that becoming a PA is my best option. I've considered becoming a nurse practitioner, but I am not currently a nurse and it would take six to eight years to accomplish this goal. I would have to attend nursing school for three or four years, get clinical experience as a nurse, and then attend nurse practitioner school for two years. Additionally, it appears that the trend for NPs is to achieve a doctorate degree, which requires even more time in school.

I've also considered becoming a physician, but given my current age and stage in life, I do not want to spend the eight-plus years it would take to become a physician, complete a two-year fellowship, and then be swamped in debt for $300,000 or more.

I do not want to become a nurse, because I have a strong desire to diagnose and treat patients.

The logical conclusion I've come to is that becoming a PA is my best option to practice medicine; I can complete PA school in two years and become part of a growing profession that offers job growth and diversity.

After joining the American Academy of Physician Assistants (AAPA) and my state chapter of the AAPA, the Connecticut Association of Physician Assistants (ConnAPA), I've been able to learn so much more about the PA profession, and I've even had the opportunity to shadow several PAs in my state.

I meet all of the prerequisite requirements to attend PA school, and I've come to the definitive conclusion that I want to become a physician assistant.

Notice how this answer is much more specific in conveying why this applicant wants to become a physician assistant. The applicant wants to practice medicine, which rules out nursing and all professions that are not medically related. The applicant rules out becoming a physician or nurse practitioner for the reasons listed above. The applicant developed a thorough understanding of the PA profession through working in a clinic as a medical assistant, joining the AAPA and ConnAPA, and shadowing several PAs in her state. She also has the required prerequisites and a strong science GPA in undergraduate school, showing she has the academic ability to complete the rigorous didactic phase of PA school. The applicant's answers address several of the scoring criteria listed in the previous chapter for PA school selection.

So think about your own answer to the question of what motivates you to specifically choose the physician assistant profession, and be sure it answers that question and you have supported your answer with relative examples. I suggest you have a friend or two also read your essay and give you feedback.

After writing your essay or preparing your answer to the question "Why do you want to become a physician assistant?" check to see if you've answered these four criteria listed below. By completing this exercise, you will have a much better chance of writing a great essay and increase your chances of being invited for an interview.

Exercise: Why do you want to become a physician assistant?

1. How will you describe that you have a thorough understanding of the PA profession? How did you obtain this knowledge? Use the space below to jot down some brief answers:

    a. _____

    b. _____

    c. _____

    d. _____

2. In your answer to the question regarding why you want to become a PA, how is your answer unique to becoming a PA versus becoming a nurse, nurse practitioner, or physician?

   a. _____

   b. _____

   c. _____

   d. _____

3. What have you done to demonstrate your passion for becoming a PA?

   a. _____

   b. _____

   c. _____

   d. _____

4. How have you demonstrated maturity?

   a. _____

   b. _____

   c. _____

   d. _____

Invest the time *now* to answer these questions. If you can't provide reasonable answers, you have revealed areas of weakness that you must work on to become a strong PA school applicant.

Now take the time to answer the rest of the questions used as scoring criteria to grade you as an applicant:

5. What is your GPA (overall and in the sciences)? _____

6. What are your GRE scores? _____

7. How have you demonstrated the ability to handle stress?

   a. _____

   b. _____

   c. _____

   d. _____

8. Why are you a good fit for the program(s) you're applying to? Use bullet points. If the answer isn't clear to you right now, come back to this question after reading the next few chapters, which explore this topic further. I also help you focus in on the answer to this question in my book *How to "Ace" the Physician Assistant School Interview*.

   a. _____

   b. _____

   c. _____

   d. _____

9. What does credibility mean to you, and how have you demonstrated this in your background?

   a. _____

   b. _____

   c. _____

   d. _____

10. How do you create trust with people and patients?

    a. _____

    b. _____

    c. _____

    d. _____

11. How do you demonstrate likeability in your daily life and with patients?

   _____

   _____

   _____

   _____

   _____

   _____

   _____

   _____

CHAPTER 3

Selecting a PA Program

WHAT DO PA PROGRAMS LOOK FOR IN A COMPETITIVE APPLICANT?

As mentioned in the previous chapter, you're most likely to be evaluated in eleven specific areas when you apply to a PA program. The exercise below is meant to help you use your answers from the previous chapter and refine your answers to the top six scoring criteria, which include a

- ▸ passion for the PA profession;
- ▸ academic ability and test scores;
- ▸ health care experience;
- ▸ understanding of the PA profession;
- ▸ maturity;
- ▸ ability to handle stress.

Passion for the PA Profession

Passion cannot be quantified. Passion, or the lack thereof, can make or break your chances of getting accepted to PA school. Applicants can demonstrate passion by having a thorough understanding of the PA profession and by accomplishing prerequisites above and beyond the average applicant.

Exercise: How have you demonstrated passion for becoming a PA?

List five things you've done to demonstrate your passion for becoming a PA. Examples might include shadowing experiences, medical experience, additional coursework to raise your GPA, joining the AAPA and your state chapter of the AAPA, etc.

1. _____
2. _____
3. _____
4. _____
5. _____

Academic Ability and Test Scores

▶ Approximately 83 percent of PA school applicants have a bachelor's degree.

▶ Approximately 50 percent of PA school applicants have a degree in biology.

Exercise: Document your GPA and GRE scores

What is your GPA?	
Overall undergraduate	
Undergraduate science	
CASPA biology, chemistry, physics	
Undergraduate non-science	

What are your GRE scores?	
Verbal reasoning	
Quantitative reasoning	
Analytical writing	

Medical Experience

Exercise: Document your health-care experience

Patient contact experience	
Other health-care experience	
Other work experience	
Community service	
Shadowing	

Now, compare your numbers with actual first-year class statistics on age, GPA, and health care experience as reported in the thirtieth (2015) *Annual Report on Physician Assistant Educational Programs in the United States*, which can be found on the Physician Assistant Education Association's (PAEA's) website (paeaonline.org.) These data are current as of 2015; however, the reports are updated on a yearly basis and can be found on the PAEA website.

FIRST-YEAR CLASS: GRADE POINT AVERAGES

GPA Category	M	SD	Mdn	n(P)
Overall undergraduate	3.52	0.14	3.52	176
Undergraduate science	3.47	0.16	3.49	163
CASPA biology, chemistry, physics (BCP)	3.42	0.17	3.45	84
Undergraduate non-science	3.54	0.20	3.59	88

FIRST-YEAR CLASS: GRE SCORES

GRE Scores	M	SD	Mdn	n(P)
Verbal reasoning	152.2	5.32	153	59
Quantitative reasoning	152.0	3.68	152	55
Analytical writing	3.9	0.28	4.0	50

NOTE: Mean (M) is the average of data values, standard deviation (SD) is the amount of deviation from a set of data values, median (Mdn) is the midpoint of data values (half above and half below), and n(P) is the number of PA programs participating.

AVERAGE HEALTH-CARE EXPERIENCE HOURS OF MATRICULATING STUDENTS

Health-Care Experience	M	SD	Mdn	n(P)
Patient contact experience	3,100	3,006	2,325	89
Other health-care experience	1,014	943	713	30
Other work experience	2,001	1.771	1,500	21
Community service	425	480	270	32
Shadowing	144	204	88	45

MEDICAL EXPERIENCE STATISTICS FOR PA APPLICANTS

Worked in health-care before applying to PA school	79%
Worked less than one year or not at all in a health-care field	27%
Worked more than nine years in a health-care field	10%
Worked less than one year or not at all in a health-care field with direct-patient contact	35%
Previously worked as a medical assistant	17%
Previously worked as an EMT/Paramedic	9%
Worked as a phlebotomist	9%
Worked as an emergency room technician	8%
Worked in medical reception/records	7%
Worked as a nurse	8%
Worked as an athletic trainer	6%
Reported "other" as previous health care experience	45%

NOTE: Respondents were permitted to indicate multiple previous health-care fields, thus the sum of all fields exceeds 100 percent.

AGE RELATED STATISTICS

First Year Class: Age	M	SD	Mdn	n(P)
Age of first-year PA student	26.1	2.51	26.0	170
Age of youngest first-year PA student	21.4	1.23	21.0	168
Age of oldest first-year PA student	44.1	7.57	44.0	168

Understanding of the PA Profession

Eighty-nine percent of respondents from the thirtieth (2015) *Annual Report on Physician Assistant Educational Programs in the United States* knew at least one PA prior to applying to PA school.

Exercise: Circle the answer as it applies to you

Are you a member of the American Academy of Physician Assistants (AAPA)?	Yes No	Why not?
Are you a member of your state chapter of the AAPA?	Yes No	Why not?
Have you shadowed at least four PAs?	Yes No	Why not?

You can join the AAPA as an affiliate member by visiting the AAPA website at aapa.org and clicking on "Join."

You can join your state chapter of the AAPA by visiting my website, andrewrodican.com, and clicking on "Free Resources," then clicking on "AAPA Constituent Chapters" to find your state. Joining your state chapter is also a great way to find local PAs to shadow.

Maturity

Maturity is another one of those areas that can't be quantified. You should have a basic understanding of what maturity means to the admissions committee. Here are some questions they will be thinking about:

- ► Can you be empathetic yet assertive?
- ► Can you handle stress under fire?
- ► Will you know when to call for help?

- Do you exhibit good judgment?
- Can you make quick decisions?
- Are you a self-starter?
- Will you require constant supervision?

Exercise: How have you demonstrated maturity?

Answer the following questions:

1. Write down the dictionary definitions of *empathetic* and *assertive*.

   Empathetic: _____

   _____

   Assertive: _____

   _____

2. Describe a situation in which you've had to be empathetic yet assertive.

   _____

   _____

   _____

   _____

3. Describe a stressful situation that you were able to resolve.

   _____

   _____

   _____

   _____

4. Write down the dictionary definition of *judgment*.

   Judgment: _____

   _____

5. Write down the dictionary definition of *autonomous*.

   Autonomous: _____

   _____

Ability to Handle Stress

The admissions committee is interested in knowing how well you deal with stress. As a physician assistant school student, you will be under constant pressure to perform well in the classroom and during clinical rotations. When you become a physician assistant, you will be required to make difficult decisions quickly and accurately. If you plan on becoming an effective and competent PA, being able to handle stress is a must. I think the underlying question that most admissions committee members ask themselves is, Can I see this applicant caring for my mother or child in a critical situation?

During the PA school interview you will be evaluated on your ability to handle stress by how well you handle the interview. Are you calm and collected, or are you a nervous wreck? You will also be asked, directly, "Tell us about a time when you had to deal with a stressful situation." The committee will also evaluate your answer for what you consider to be a stressful situation.

I strongly recommend that you think about stressful situations you've faced in the past and write them down now.

Exercise: Examples of how you've handled stress in the past

Fill in the blanks:

EXAMPLE 1

The situation or task was: _____

_____

_____

The action I took was:_____

_____

_____

The result was: _____

_____

_____

EXAMPLE 2

The situation or task was: _____

_____

_____

The action I took was:_____

_____

_____

The result was: _____

_____

_____

EXAMPLE 3

The situation or task was: _____

_____

_____

The action I took was:_____

_____

_____

The result was: _____

_____

_____

THE TOURNAMENT DRAW TECHNIQUE

During the PA school application process, you may become overwhelmed by the number of items you will need to accomplish. Let's take a look at a common to-do list:

1. Prepare for entrance exams.
2. Take entrance exams.
3. Register for microbiology course to meet prerequisite.
4. Find four PAs to shadow.
5. Gain hands-on medical experience.
6. Draft essay.
7. Locate three people to provide letters of recommendation.
8. Join the American Academy of Physician Assistants (AAPA).
9. Join your state/constituent chapter of the AAPA.
10. Save $100 per week.
11. Speak with three program graduates.
12. Attend program open houses.
13. Speak with program directors.
14. Complete the Centralized Application Service for Physician Assistants (CASPA) application.
15. Complete microbiology course.
16. Contact volunteer offices to find medically-related volunteer work

If you have more items to include on this list, by all means include them. The following technique will work for as many items as you have in squares of two.

This technique is based on the NCAA basketball "March Madness" bracket selection. In round one all of the teams (items on your list) are placed into the initial bracket. As the team, or item, wins that team (item) moves on to the next round, until we end up with a winner. This winning item should be your first one to accomplish on your path to becoming a PA. You can work your way backward, and work more than one item at a time, until you've accomplished all of your goals. Prioritizing your list using this technique will take a lot of the anxiety and guesswork out of the application process.

If you look at the results of the exercise on the opposite page, you can see that this particular applicant needs to gain medical experience to meet the prerequisites for the PA programs she is interested in. Given this fact, the applicant's number one focus should be to find a position where she can gain some hands-on medical experience. If she cannot meet the admissions requirements/prerequisites, all of the other items become moot. I don't want to imply that applicants can't simultaneously work on some of the other items, like registering

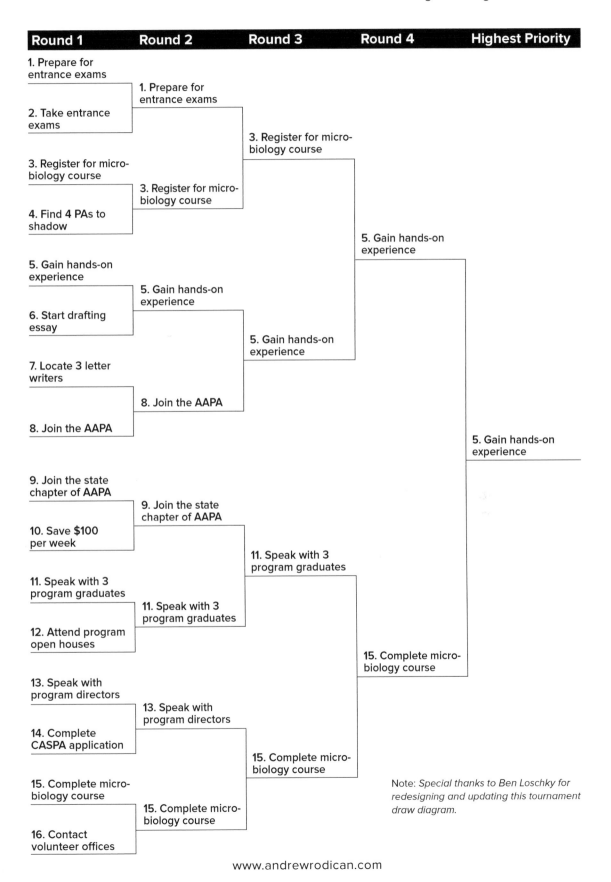

Round 1	Round 2	Round 3	Round 4	Highest Priority

1. Prepare for entrance exams

1. Prepare for entrance exams

2. Take entrance exams

3. Register for microbiology course

3. Register for microbiology course

3. Register for microbiology course

4. Find 4 PAs to shadow

5. Gain hands-on experience

5. Gain hands-on experience

5. Gain hands-on experience

6. Start drafting essay

5. Gain hands-on experience

5. Gain hands-on experience

7. Locate 3 letter writers

8. Join the AAPA

8. Join the AAPA

5. Gain hands-on experience

9. Join the state chapter of AAPA

9. Join the state chapter of AAPA

10. Save $100 per week

11. Speak with 3 program graduates

11. Speak with 3 program graduates

11. Speak with 3 program graduates

12. Attend program open houses

15. Complete microbiology course

13. Speak with program directors

13. Speak with program directors

14. Complete CASPA application

15. Complete microbiology course

15. Complete microbiology course

15. Complete microbiology course

16. Contact volunteer offices

Note: *Special thanks to Ben Loschky for redesigning and updating this tournament draw diagram.*

for a microbiology class, while gaining medical experience. In fact, applicants will more than likely need to multitask to accomplish all of these items.

Your list may be completely different. You can fill out your own tournament draw sheet to see where you stand.

Exercise: The tournament draw technique

Complete the list below using the form as a template, make a draw sheet big enough to accommodate all the items on your to-do list. There can be eight, sixteen, thirty-two, or sixty-four lines. This is the preliminary draw. Now you decide which goals are most important—that is, which ones will move you to the next round. Repeat this process until you end up with the final eight. These now have become your main draw. Repeat the procedure until you end up with a winner.

1. _____
2. _____
3. _____
4. _____
5. _____
6. _____
7. _____
8. _____
9. _____
10. _____
11. _____
12. _____
13. _____
14. _____
15. _____
16. _____

Round 1	Round 2	Round 3	Round 4	Highest Priority

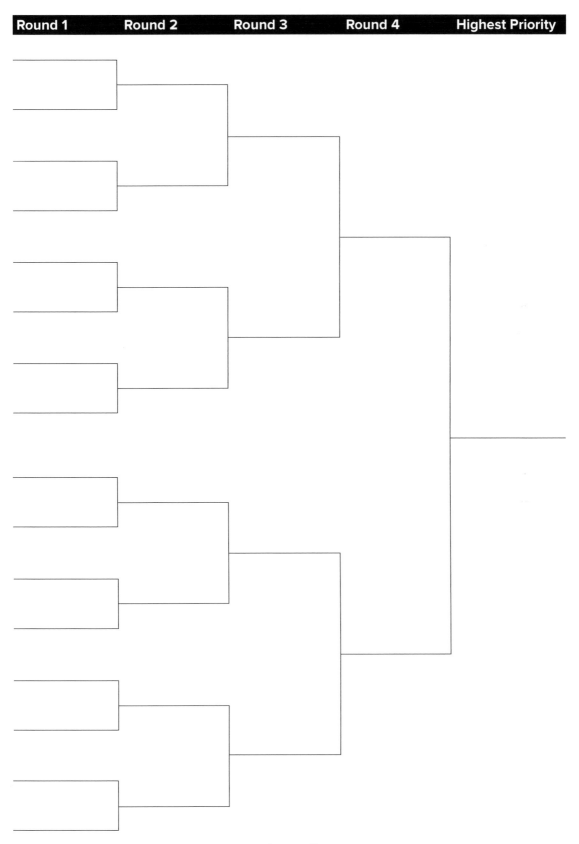

FIVE TIPS FOR SELECTING A PA PROGRAM

Due to the competitiveness of getting into PA school, many applicants feel that getting into *any* program would be just fine with them. However, there are many factors to consider when selecting a PA program, because all programs are not alike. If you choose to apply to the wrong program(s), you may be in for a rude awakening when it comes to getting a quality training experience and/or being prepared to take the certification examination (PANCE) when you graduate.

If you choose a program that is a good fit for you and a program that is well established, your chances of getting a quality education and passing your certification exam will be excellent.

Here are five tools to consider when selecting a PA program:

1. **Visit my website (andrewrodican.com), and click on "Resources" to find a listing of current PA programs.** The list contains all of the accredited PA programs in the United States. It also includes programs that are provisionally accredited and those that are seeking accreditation. Additionally, you can search for information on tuition, prerequisites, financial aid, test scores, essay requirements and content, curriculum, and clinical rotations.

2. **Check the accreditation status of the program(s).** You must make sure the program you are applying to is accredited by the Commission on Accreditation of Allied Health Education Programs. If you do not graduate from an accredited PA program, you will not be eligible to sit for the national boards (PANCE), administered by the National Commission on Certification of Physician Assistants (NCCPA).

3. **Find out the focus of the program(s).** Certain programs mention a particular focus in print literature or on the Internet. For instance, the City University of New York (CUNY) Harlem Hospital Center PA Program focuses on practice in underserved areas.

4. **Find out the program's first-time pass/fail rate on the NCCPA certification examination.** I stress the *first-time* pass/fail rate on the NCCPA exam, because if you don't ask the program representatives in those specific terms, you will get the *overall* pass/fail rate; eventually most students pass. Look for a program with a first-time pass/fail rate in the mid to high 90th percentile. This number is usually listed on the program's website.

5. **Set up meetings with the program director and some students.**
   Set up a one-on-one meeting with the program director. This is a great opportunity to learn more about the program and demonstrate your passion for the PA profession. It is also a good idea to make contact with some of the students. Find out what they like and don't like about the program. This information can be invaluable at the interview. There are PA student societies at many programs, which you can find online.

CHAPTER 4

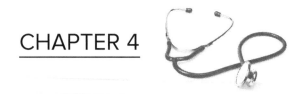

Completing Your Personal Goal Sheet

"Whatever we think about and thank about we bring about."

—John Demartini

The story goes like this: It was the bottom of the ninth inning during a World Series baseball game. The pitching coach came to the mound and had a conversation with his pitcher. You see, the batter was the best hitter on the opposing team. The bases were loaded, and this imposing batter represented the winning run. "Whatever you do, don't pitch him low and inside," the pitching coach said before walking back to the dugout.

The pitcher went into his windup and threw the pitch, and . . . you guessed it, the pitch was *low and inside*. The result was a game-winning grand slam.

What does this have to do with the topic, you ask? When that pitching coach left the mound, the only thing the pitcher remembered was *low and inside*. We bring about what we think about. If the pitching coach had said, "Pitch him high and outside," the results may have been much different.

Our subconscious mind doesn't have any filters. It will deliver to us anything we ask of it. It's also a storehouse of knowledge. Have you ever been in the middle of a conversation and been unable to remember an acquaintance's name? You grit your teeth and say, "It's right on the tip of my tongue," and then continue talking about other things. Then, all of a sudden, you remember, *Mary Smith*! What you did was turn over to your subconscious mind the order to find that name in its data bank. Sure enough, your subconscious delivered.

If you focus on how competitive it is to get into PA school and if you don't believe at a subconscious level that you can accomplish this worthy goal, you're right! If you focus on the fact that you're an excellent candidate and you will get into the PA school of your choice, you're also right!

I bargained with Life for a penny,
And Life would pay no more;
However I begged at evening
When I counted my scanty store.

For Life is a just employer;
He gives you what you ask,
But once you have set the wages,
Why, you must bear the task.

I worked for a menial's hire,
Only to learn, dismayed,
That any wage I had asked of Life,
Life would have willingly paid.

—Jesse B. Rittenhouse

As I mention in my original best-selling book, *The Ultimate Guide to Getting into Physician Assistant School*, I am a huge believer in imaging: seeing the goal accomplished in my head before I achieve it. I've used a picture board to help focus on all of my goals for the future; my bucket list. One of my main goals after retirement is to travel the country in an RV and visit every national park and monument in the United States. I also want to travel to Rome and Paris. On my picture board I have a photo of the RV I want to buy, pictures of national parks and monuments, pictures of the Roman Colosseum and the Eiffel Tower, and a map of all of the states. I have this board in my living room and add to it as I develop new goals.

When I was applying to PA school, my number one choice was Yale. I lived in New Haven, I had two small children, my ex-wife had a solid job in New Haven, and the program was well established, with a great reputation. There were many other reasons why I wanted to attend Yale. What I did was get an envelope with the Yale PA program's logo on it. I leaned it against a TV in my bedroom, and every day I would work out on my NordicTrack and visualize myself going to the mailbox, opening the letter, and reading the word "Congratulations." As I did this every day, I noticed my heart rate increasing, and a smile would come to my face as I actually *felt* how great it was going to feel opening that letter.

I accomplished that goal!

I suggest that you do a similar thing—either with a picture board, letterhead, or logo of your number one program. Then complete exercises that follow later in the chapter and you'll be well on your way to achieving your goal of getting into the PA school of your choice.

SEVEN-STEP FORMULA FOR SUCCESS

"Whatever the mind of man can conceive and believe it can achieve."
—NAPOLEON HILL (*Think and Grow Rich*)

The following seven-step formula for success will help you accomplish any worthy goal in life:

1. Identify the goal.
2. Set a deadline for achievement.
3. List obstacles to overcome.
4. Identify people and organizations that can help you.
5. List the skills and knowledge required to achieve your goal.
6. Develop a plan of action.
7. List the benefits of achieving the goal, and ask yourself, "What do I have to gain?"

Here is my original goal sheet from August 15, 1990:

By May 1, 1992, I will be accepted into the Yale University School of Medicine Physician Associate program, University of Florida, or Bowman Gray's Physician Assistant Program. In order to accomplish this goal, I will first have to discuss my desire to become a PA with my wife and convince her that this is the right thing to do for our family. Next, I will need to begin saving money so that I can help my wife support our two children and provide food and shelter for the next two years. Finally, I will stay focused and not listen to those people who will say I'm crazy or having an early midlife crisis for wanting to quit a great job at age thirty-five and go back to school for two years.

I will immediately contact the American Academy of Physician Assistants and the Connecticut Academy of Physician Assistants (Conn-APA) to find out what resources are available to me. I will initiate contact with all three of my desired programs. I will contact the president of Conn-APA and get to know him. I will also visit Yale's PA program, meet with the dean of the program, and maintain contact with her quarterly. I will find out what I lack as a competitive candidate and how I can best strengthen my application.

I will visit with some PAs who work in my wife's office and spend as much time with them as possible (shadowing). I will attend Yale's open house to learn more about the program, speak with students, and make myself known to them.

I will need anatomy and physiology (I and II) and microbiology to fulfill requirements (prerequisites). I will achieve no less than an A in each class. I will also begin volunteering at Saint Raphael's hospital, in the ER, in order to gain more current experience. I will also obtain an SAT study guide to prepare myself for the test, which I need to take to apply to Yale.

My plan is to continue working full time, save money, and do volunteer work part time. I will also take evening classes. While working in a hospital, I will discuss my goals with as many PAs as possible and learn as much as I can about the PA profession.

Once I achieve my goal of getting into the PA school of my choice, I will enjoy many benefits: helping people, job satisfaction, a secure future, challenging and stimulating work, prestige, a sense of accomplishment, and much more.

GOAL ACCOMPLISHED

Fast-forward to 2015. I'm a 1994 graduate of the Yale University Physician Associate Program. Since graduating, I have worked in five specialty areas: cardiothoracic surgery, occupational medicine, cardiology, bariatric medicine (in which I owned my own clinic for eight years), and family practice/internal medicine. I've authored four books for PA school applicants: *The Ultimate Guide to Getting into Physician Assistant School, How to "Ace" the Physician Assistant School Interview, Essays That Will Get You into Physician Assistant School,* and this current workbook. Even now, I still utilize goal sheets to help me fulfill my other dreams and passions in life.

Before you create your own goal sheet, I want you to complete the following exercise. It will take a little time to do the research but will be well worth it. (Visit the "Resources" section of my website, andrewrodican.com, for access to an updated and comprehensive list of all PA schools in the United States.)

Exercise: Selecting PA programs to apply to

Fill in the blanks relative to your top five choices of PA programs. The first grid is a sample of what your own might look like.

PA Program	Program Focus	1st Time Pass/Fail Rate	All Prerequisites Met?
Emory	No	99%	Yes
University of Alabama-Birmingham	Surgery	97%	Yes
University of Utah	Underserved and rural communities	94%	No
Trevecca Nazarene	Integrating faith in learning by educating from a Christian worldview	93%	Yes
Quinnipiac University	No	98.3%	Yes
Notes:			

If we look at the chart, we can eliminate two of the programs immediately: University of Utah (prerequisites aren't met) and, assuming you don't want to be a surgical PA, University of Alabama.

Now let's look at the rest. Unless you're particularly religious, your odds of getting accepted to Trevecca are slim. Emory and Quinnipiac are good choices for you because they have no particular focus and you've met the prerequisites.

I recommend that you do this exercise for every program you plan to apply to. It will give you a clearer picture of what programs may be a good fit for your goals and résumé. If you've been able to eliminate any of your choices after realistically looking at your results, add in other programs to complete your list.

PA Program	Program Focus	1st Time Pass/Fail Rate	All Prerequisites Met?
Notes:			

Now it's time to complete your own personal goal sheet for getting into the PA school of your choice. You should now have enough information to decide on your top choice. Fill in the blanks, laminate the sheet, and read it every night before you go to bed and every morning when you wake up.

Exercise: List your top five PA programs

1. _____

2. _____

3. _____

4. _____

5. _____

Exercise: Identify your goal and set a deadline for achievement

I will be accepted to the _____ PA Program

by _____ 20_____.

Exercise: List obstacles to overcome

1. _____
2. _____
3. _____
4. _____
5. _____
6. _____
7. _____
8. _____
9. _____
10. _____

Exercise: Identify people and organizations that can help you

A few examples are listed below:

1. AJR Associates (Andy Rodican, PA-C)
2. The American Academy of Physician Assistants
3. My state chapter of the AAPA
4. _____
5. _____
6. _____

7. _____

8. _____

9. _____

10. _____

Exercise: List the skills and knowledge required to achieve your goal

1. _____

2. _____

3. _____

4. _____

5. _____

Exercise: Develop a plan of action

_____

_____

_____

_____

_____

_____

_____

_____

_____

_____

Exercise: List the benefits of achieving this goal. What do you hope to gain?

Examples are listed below.

1. Excellent job-growth potential

2. Ability to practice medicine

3. _____

4. _____

5. _____

Exercise: Complete your own goal sheet

Write out your own goal sheet based on the above information. Laminate the sheet and place it somewhere where you will read it every night before going to bed and every morning upon awakening.

Date: __ __ / __ __ / __ __ __ __

_____

_____

_____

_____

_____

_____

_____

_____

_____

_____

_____

_____

_____

CHAPTER 5

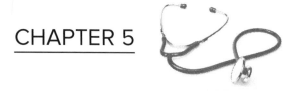

The Application Process

For the vast majority of PA school applicants, the process of applying to PA school will start with the Central Application Service for Physician Assistants (CASPA) application.

BACKGROUND ON THE CASPA APPLICATION

In 1991, I applied to three PA programs; Yale, University of Florida, and Wake Forest. Each program had its own application forms and application fees. I probably invested over six hundred dollars (or more) applying to these three schools. Each of these three programs also had unique requirements relative to prerequisites, health care experience, GPA, and essay questions. If you wanted to apply individually to ten PA programs in 1991, you would have to accomplish ten separate applications along with the accompanying fees. The process was costly and extremely time consuming.

In 2001, the Physician Assistant Education Association (PAEA) began using the first centralized application service for physician assistant school applicants—the Central Application Service for Physician Assistants (CASPA.) This service allows applicants to complete a single online application, and will send this application to any PA program designated by the applicant. In 2016, the cost for a CASPA application is $175, and $50 dollars for each additional program that utilizes the CASPA application.

Not all PA programs participate with CASPA, and you will need to accomplish separate applications for these schools.

Currently, applicants can obtain detailed information about the CASPA application at https://help.unicas.com:88/caspahelpPages/about-caspaoverview /index.html and on the CASPA website at https://portal.caspaonline.org. These addresses may change in the future, so I recommend using a search engine and plug in "Central Application Service for Physician Assistants Application" if these sites aren't valid at the time of your application.

BENEFITS OF THE CASPA APPLICATION

Since 2001, I've coached thousands of PA school applicants and reviewed hundreds of CASPA applications. I've listened to the applicants' feedback on the application process and why they like using this service. Here are some of the benefits they appreciate most:

1. The ability to apply to multiple PA programs using a single online application.
2. The checklist and instructions provided on the CASPA website, which simplifies the accomplishment of the CASPA application.
3. The fact that they only have to provide transcripts, letters of recommendation, health care experience hours, and demographic data once. They do not have to gather and repeat this data for each program they apply to.
4. The ability to access their CASPA application from any computer and update and save data right up until the time they actually submit their application.

PAY STRICT ATTENTION TO DETAIL WHEN ACCOMPLISHING YOUR CASPA APPLICATION

At first glance, the CASPA application looks extremely intimidating. There is so much information to gather and so many deadlines to meet before an application is considered complete. But don't worry, if you methodically go through the instructions and complete one task at a time, you will make it to the finish line. Think about how many of your predecessors completed this application and believe that you can do it too.

The most valuable piece of advice I can provide to you is to make sure that you follow instructions and pay strict attention to detail. After all, these are the traits of a good PA. I know that you'll be excited to get the application process started and completed, but if you rush and don't pay attention to every detail you will regret it later. Here is an example of what I mean:

> *After graduating from college in 1984, I made the decision to become an air force officer. I signed up with a recruiter, and headed off to Officer Training School (OTS) in San Antonio, Texas. OTS was an intense twelve week program. In order to complete the program, we had to pass certain "measurements", or physical, academic, and military bearing requirements, during the twelve week process. If you failed three measurements along the way, you were discharged from the air force.*

In the first week, I had to complete a measurement in the form of a simple test. We had only five minutes to complete 50 questions. Looking at the test, the sheer volume of questions and the strict time limit placed on us made me extremely anxious. I didn't want to fail a measurement in my first week.

The proctor advised us that we could begin immediately after he said "Start", and when he said "Stop", we were to drop our pencils immediately. My heart was racing as he then said, "Start."

I noticed a small paragraph at the top of the first page and after a quick glance; I decided the information was just a repeat of what he told us before the exam began. I didn't want to waste any time. With sweaty palms, I quickly began reading and answering the questions. I started to relax when I realized the questions were very basic and easy to answer. I thought to myself, "piece of cake." It almost seemed too simple.

After I realized I was going to finish the exam with plenty of time to spare, I began to relax and I happened to look up at some of the other candidates. Some were feverishly answering the questions, and some were sitting still in their seats not doing anything. I looked at them curiously and initially thought that perhaps they already finished the exam.

Then I started to get a little knot in my stomach. Something wasn't right. I went on to complete the exam and finished in plenty of time. The proctor said "Stop", and I was confident I had done well. Then he spoke the words that I will never forget, "Those of you who answered any of the questions on this exam failed this measurement." My heart sank, and I went into panic mode. Why is he saying this? He then went on to read that paragraph (paraphrased) at the top of the page:

> This measurement is to be completed in five minutes. Be sure to read all of the questions carefully. Once the proctor says start, you will have five minutes to complete the exam. Do not answer any of the questions or check any of the boxes.

Now it made sense why some of the candidates were sitting still; they read that first paragraph in its entirety and I simply glanced over it to save time.

So I flunked my first measurement in my first week of training. If I failed two more measurements in the next eleven weeks I was out.

I learned a valuable lesson that day; always pay strict attention to detail! Failure to pay strict attention to detail in the military can lead to a loss of life and failing to pay strict attention to detail on your CASPA application can lead to a rejection letter from the PA school(s) you are applying to.

SEVEN TIPS FOR USING THE CASPA APPLICATION

Here are some tips to follow before and during the process of accomplishing the CASPA application:

1. Follow instructions. Be sure to read all of the instructions on the CASPA application prior to submitting it.

2. Be sure to know exactly who you will need to obtain letters of recommendation from; a physician, a physician assistant, a supervisor, a professor, etc.

3. Be sure to request all of your transcripts early and have them sent directly to you. This will help you accomplish the course-work portion of the application.

4. Be sure that your essay does not exceed the 5000 character limit. If your essay is more than 5000 characters it will be cut off. Make sure that your essay is error free. Read the essay backwards to catch spelling errors; read the essay from the last word in the last paragraph to the first word in the first paragraph. By using this technique you will find that spelling errors will pop right out at you. Also, be sure to have your essay reviewed for spelling and grammar before you submit it. One spelling or grammatical error can spell disaster.

5. Make sure that you meet the deadlines for all of the programs that you are applying to, because each program has its own deadline.

6. Make sure you visit the websites of the programs you are applying to, and be sure that you meet, or exceed, all of the requirements if you want to be a competitive applicant.

7. Apply Early. Register as soon as you decide to apply to PA school, and try to get your CASPA application in several weeks before each programs' deadline. Start acquiring the following information that you will need to accomplish the application:

   a. A complete accounting of your health care experience, including job descriptions, number of hours accumulated, and dates of employment. Document dates and duties of all volunteer experiences and shadowing experiences.

   b. Obtain a personal copy of required test scores.

   c. Collect copies of any certificates that you may have earned, including awards, certifications, and any specialized training you may have completed.

    d. Decide whom you will choose to write your letters of recommendation (see chapter 6 for specifics.) Be sure to ask people who know you well and you feel confident that they will write a positive recommendation and will submit it on time.

SAMPLE APPLICATION TIMELINE

Here is a sample timeline used to apply to a hypothetical PA program with an application due by September 1 of the following year.

September 1, 20XX to October 1, 20XX

- Purchase a copy of my book, *The Ultimate Guide to Getting Into Physician Assistant School*, and read it thoroughly.
- Research several PA programs online.
- Decide which programs you would like to attend.
- Accomplish your personal goal sheet as discussed in chapter 4.
- Use the exercises in chapter 3 to see how competitive an applicant you will be at each program.
- Write down your final list of programs after completing your research.
- Become familiar with the CASPA application website.
- Continue accumulating health care experience.
- Register for any classes that you may need to retake or accomplish to meet prerequisites.

October 2, 20XX to November 1, 20XX

- Begin the CASPA application process by going to the CASPA website and clicking on "My Application." Obtain a username and password and begin filling in your personal information. You will now be able to return to your application at any time and continue to complete the various sections.
- Order the required transcripts from each college you've attended.
- Begin thinking about three people whom you can approach to write strong letters of recommendation in support of your candidacy.
- Write the first draft of your essay.
- Open a bank account and start saving as much money as you can to help with tuition, books, or medical equipment.

November 2, 20XX to December 1, 20XX:

- ▶ Call each program that you are applying to and ask if they have open house events for applicants.
- ▶ Try to get a one-on-one consultation with the program director or any other staff member at the programs.
- ▶ Place the dates of the open houses in your calendar and plan to attend some or all of them. Make it a point to attend your three top choice programs' open house.
- ▶ Join the American Academy of Physician Assistants (AAPA) and your state chapter of the AAPA as an affiliate member.
- ▶ Visit the AAPA website and your state chapter's website often. Focus on current events, information relevant to applicants and any meetings that you may be able to attend in order to network and meet potential PAs to shadow.
- ▶ Write a second draft of your essay.
- ▶ Join the PA Forum and begin following the threads related to pre-physician assistants, physician assistant students, CASPA, and personal statements. Read through the posts, and post your own questions that you would like answered. Continue following the PA Forum right up until your interview.
- ▶ Check the websites of your selected PA programs and inquire if they have a PA student society. See if you can network with any of the students who belong.

December 2, 20XX to January 1, 20XX

- ▶ Take a breather for the holiday season.
- ▶ Continue following the PA Forum, and visiting the AAPA and your state chapter of the AAPA websites.
- ▶ Begin thinking about PAs to shadow and any volunteer work that you can find.

January 2, 20XX to February 1, 20XX

- ▶ Secure three shadowing opportunities with local PAs
- ▶ Sign up for a GRE course, if you haven't already taken the test.
- ▶ Start attending open houses for your selected programs.

February 2, 20XX to March 1, 20XX

- ► Take the GREs
- ► Begin shadowing PAs
- ► Begin volunteer work

March 2, 20XX to April 1, 20XX

- ► Continue using all of the resources available to you and make it your job to be an expert on the PA profession.
- ► Continue shadowing and volunteering.
- ► Update your CASPA application as needed.
- ► Secure three people to write letters of recommendation for you.

April 2, 20XX to May 1, 20XX

- ► Ask the people who are writing your letters of recommendation if you can supply them with bullet points, or better yet, a completed letter of recommendation.
- ► Write your own letters of recommendation and/or bullet points; refer to chapter 6.
- ► Continue checking your CASPA application status.

May 2, 20XX to June 1, 20XX

- ► Continue to follow the PA Forum and ask any specific questions that you may still have pertaining to your selected programs or pertaining to the PA profession.
- ► Continue to follow current events on the AAPA website and your state chapter of the AAPA website.
- ► Monitor your application status.

June 2, 20XX to July 1, 20XX

- ► Complete the Colleges Attended section and the References section immediately so that references and transcripts can be received by CASPA.
- ► Request that transcripts be sent to CASPA directly from your schools and confirm with your references that they have received the online reference request via e-mail. Request that additional copies of

transcripts be sent to you directly so that you may begin entering your coursework into your CASPA application. Write the third draft of your personal essay.

July 2, 20XX to August 1, 20XX

▶ Monitor application for receipt of transcripts and letters of reference and follow up with CASPA on any missing items. Complete filling out your application and submit it to CASPA.

August 2, 20XX to September 1, 20XX

▶ CASPA application has been submitted and all transcripts, payments, and at least two letters of reference have posted to the CASPA application. The application has received a complete date and is in line for verification. Monitor your application status regularly and follow up on any incomplete or undelivered statuses until the application is "verified."

September 2, 20XX to Interview Date

▶ Purchase my book, *How to Ace the Physician Assistant School Interview,* and begin learning about the interview process and the types of interview questions that you will be asked.

▶ Have a friend or family member ask you the interview questions in my book and practice, practice, practice.

▶ Start visualizing yourself receiving your invitation to interview. Visualize yourself doing well at the interview and keep visualizing that scenario every day.

▶ Congratulate yourself for doing a fantastic job!

APPLICATION STATUS AND NOTIFICATIONS

CASPA will not email you if you have any incomplete data in your file. You must be proactive and frequently check the status of your application on a regular basis. The last thing you want to discover a week before your deadline is that one of your reference letters hasn't been submitted.

To check the status of your application at any given time, open your CASPA application and click on the "Manage My Programs " tab, then click on "Program Status."

The following is a list of statuses you may encounter:

1. In Progress
2. Received—Awaiting Materials
3. Materials Received—Verifying
4. Complete Date
5. Complete Date Currently Being Verified
6. Undelivered
7. Verfied

HOW DOES CASPA CALCULATE MY GPA?

CASPA automatically performs the following steps when calculating your GPA: This process is not done manually. The calculation utilizes "Quality Points" (QP), letter grade of each course, semester hours of each course, and cumulative attempted hours for all courses.

CASPA Formula:

Number of Credit Hours × Letter Grade = Quality Points
Number of Quality Points/Total Credit Hours = Calculated GPA

CASPA breaks down your GPA by course subject, regardless of your college level. These subjects are determined by the "CASPA course subjects" you selected for each course on your application. Please note that during the verification process, CASPA staff will change the subject category for any courses which they determine were not categorized correctly.

Course Subject GPAs

Course	Graded Credits	QP	GPA
Biology/Zoology	84.0	270.0	3.21
Inorganic Chemistry	6.0	15.0	2.50
Organic Chemistry	6.0	18.0	3.00
Biochemistry	12.0	31.8	2.65
Physics	6.0	13.8	2.30
BCP Totals	**114.0**	**348.6**	**3.06**
Other Science	3.0	12.0	4.00
Math	15.0	40.8	2.72
English	12.0	43.8	3.65
Behavioral Science	15.0	45.6	3.04
Other Non-Science	8.0	26.9	3.36
Total	**167.0**	**517.7**	**3.10**

CASPA breaks down your GPA by school year, and also divides your courses into Science, Non-Science, and Overall categories.

Year-Level GPAs

Category	Science			Non-Science			Total		
	Credits	QP	GPA	Credits	QP	GPA	Credits	QP	GPA
Freshman	18.0	60.9	3.38	15.0	50.7	3.38	33.0	83.1	2.52
Sophomore	18.0	49.8	2.77	6.0	9.9	1.65	24.0	59.7	2.49
Junior	18.0	60.9	3.38	15.0	50.7	3.38	33.0	11.6	3.38
Senior	30.0	84.6	2.82	0.0	0.0	0.00	30.0	84.6	2.82
Total	84.0	256.2	2.83	36.0	10.1	2.81	120.0	339.0	2.82
Post-Baccalaureate	3.0	12.0	4.0	11.0	44.0	4.00	14.0	56.0	4.00
Cumulative Undergraduate	87.0	249.9	2.87	47.0	145.1	3.09	134.0	395.0	2.95
Graduate	30.0	110.7	3.69	3.0	12.0	4.00	33.0	122.7	3.72
Doctorate	0.0	0.0	0.00	0.0	0.0	0.00	00.0	0.0	0.00
Overall	117.0	360.6	3.08	50.0	157.1	3.14	167.0	517.7	3.10

Letter Grade CASPA Values

Grade on Transcript	CASPA Letter Grade	CASPA Numeric Value
A+	A	4.0
A	A	4.0
A-	A-	3.7
AB	AB	3.5
B+	B+	3.3
B	B	3.0
B-	B-	2.7
BC	BC	2.5
C+	C+	2.3
C	C	2.0
C-	C-	1.7
CD	CD	1.5
D+	D+	1.3
D	D	1.0
D-	D-	0.7
E	E	0.0
WF	WF	0.0

CASPA CONTACT INFORMATION

Customer Service:	(617) 612-2800
	Open Monday–Friday 9:00 a.m.–5:00 p.m. EST
Customer Service E-mail:	caspainfo@caspaonline.
CASPA Facebook Page:	http://facebook.com/CASPAOnlineApp
CASPA Twitter Feed:	https://twitter.com/CASPAOnlineApp

SUPPLEMENTAL APPLICATIONS

Some programs require applicants to complete a supplemental application in addition to the CASPA application. Yes, more work. However, I recommend that you view the supplemental application as an opportunity, rather than a nuisance. The supplemental questions will give you more insight into what the program is looking for in qualified applicants. The more you can learn about a program, the better your chances of succeeding at the interview.

This is one example of what a supplemental application may look like:

SAMPLE SUPPLEMENTAL APPLICATION

1. Instructions: Complete the supplemental application and e-mail it to the program's email address. Use your last name and first name as the file name (e.g. Smith John).

2. Please provide the following required information:

   Name _____

   Street _____

   City _____

   E-mail _____

   Home Phone _____   Cell Phone _____

3. Are you state resident?   Yes   No

   If yes, length of residency: _____

4. Are any of your relatives alumni of our program?   Yes   No

5. Have you previously applied to our program?   Yes   No

6. Have you previously been interviewed at our program?   Yes   No

---

CASPA applications are not considered complete and will not be reviewed until the required supplemental application and online fee are received by the program.

Please answer the following questions in 250 words or less:

1. What three attributes of our program most influenced you to apply to our program and why?
2. Other than becoming a competent medical provider, discuss two other skills that you hope to learn as a student in our program?
3. Do you consider yourself to be a role model? If so, to whom and why?
4. Based on your clinical experience, identify a health care challenge you have encountered. Describe specific steps you initiated to overcome this obstacle and the impact this had on patient care outcomes.
5. Describe your experience caring for medically underserved populations and its impact on your goals as a future health care provider.
6. List any leadership positions or roles you have assumed and discuss how these experiences have influenced your leadership style.

Please carefully read and consider the following. Then sign electronically in the space indicated.

- Any falsification of information provided by an applicant related to his/her CASPA or supplemental applications will result in the nullification of an interview offer and/or offer of admission.
- Felony and Misdemeanor Conviction Disclosure Statement

Many of the clinical affiliates that are utilized by our require background checks of any student who will be interacting with patients or who rotate through their facility. Therefore, all students admitted to our program are required to complete a criminal background check and provide the program with the final report no later than May 1, 20XX. Instructions will be provided to those candidates offered seats after they have indicated that they accept an offer of admission to our program. Failure to provide a copy of the criminal background check by the May 1, 20XX deadline will result in automatic rescission of any offer of admission.

I have read the statements above and agree to the terms specified. I explicitly acknowledge that I must obtain a criminal background check if I am offered a seat in the program and understand that if I admitted I am required to provide the program with a copy of the results of said criminal background check from the agency specified by our program by no later than May 1, 20XX.

_____   _____

Signature   Date

So here is the opportunity: take a look at the first two questions and you'll realize that the answer to these questions are very important to this program. What are the correct answers to these questions? Just look at the mission statement, vision statement, and objectives of the program on its website and you'll find the answers.

For question number one, I suggest looking at the program's page on their website. You'll find many attributes of the program listed right there, such as

- a five-year (first-time) PANCE pass rate for the program of 98 percent, national 93 percent;
- a student-to-faculty ratio of nine to one;
- the third ranked public research university in the United States.

You can use these three attributes as topic sentences for your 250-word answer to question number 1.

For question number two, look at the "About our Program" page:

The school is committed to educating and preparing its students to practice at the forefront of a dynamic healthcare system. Focusing on a team approach to healthcare, students from all programs enroll in core classes and work together on group projects. This allows students to understand the collaboration necessary to provide quality, effective healthcare.

The campus-based degree programs combine comprehensive didactic education with practical experience. Students train in over 500 state and national clinical sites in a variety of rural and urban settings (hospitals, clinics, private practices, and rehabilitation centers). This experience encourages the development of interpersonal skills, knowledge, and practical application.

1. You will learn with a team approach and work with other students on group projects.

2. You will work in a variety of rural and urban settings

3. You will graduate with the education and knowledge to practice in the forefront of a dynamic healthcare system.

As you can see, programs proudly publish this material on their websites. This is also valuable information that you must know when you have an interview at the school. The rest of the questions require answers based on your personal background and will not be found on any website.

CHAPTER 6

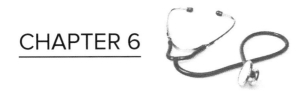

The Letter of Recommendation

Obtaining a strong letter of recommendation (LOR) may be just one of many pieces needed to fit into the PA program application puzzle, but missing this one critical piece can spell disaster. On the other hand, a perfect fit—a strong letter written by the right candidate—may compensate for some less relevant or weaker components.

It has been my experience over the many years I've coached PA school applicants and served on admissions committees that many candidates choose the wrong people to write a letter of recommendation. Choose people who know you well enough and understand your goal of becoming a PA. These people will be able to comment specifically on the attributes you have that will make you a great PA student and eventually a great PA.

Be wary of asking a person you think has a great reputation in the PA world or in the local community—the Big Shot. These people tend to be extremely busy, and writing your letter of recommendation is probably not their top priority. You may find yourself panicking if the deadline is near and they haven't submitted your letter of recommendation yet. Now what do you do?

If you don't believe me about all of this, just log on to the PA forums for pre-physician assistants and read some of the frantic posts about not having the LOR submitted with the deadline quickly approaching. "What should I do?" they ask. Well, the best medicine is always preventive medicine. Unfortunately, when applicants don't put a lot of thought into this process, the result may be an incomplete application.

Additionally, when asking people to write letters of recommendation, be sure to ask for exactly what you want: "Do you feel that you can write a strong and positive letter of recommendation for me?" They may say no if you put the question this way, saving you from embarrassment at the interview when you find out they didn't exactly write a glowing recommendation letter. If they agree, they've knowingly agreed to write a great LOR.

This chapter will help you obtain killer LORs that will be submitted on time and are guaranteed to be strong, persuasive letters supporting your candidacy for PA school.

FOUR MUSTS FOR OBTAINING A POWERFUL LETTER OF RECOMMENDATION

1. Know *how* to ask for it.

If you ask people to write letters of recommendation for you, they will likely agree. However, are they simply being polite, feeling obliged, or will they really have a desire to happily write them for you? If you ask for a recommendation in the way I described above, you will have a much better chance of success. Here's a suggestion: "Professor Jones, I am applying to PA school, and I would like to know if you would feel comfortable writing a *strong and favorable* letter of recommendation for me?"

2. Know *whom* to ask for it.

The strongest letters of recommendation come from those who know you well enough to make specific comments on you as a person and your abilities as a professional. This is a better criterion than selecting a Big Shot or seeking absolutely anyone just to fill this square on the CASPA application.

3. Know *what's* in it.

How do you accomplish this? Write the letter yourself! That's right, if you write the letter of recommendation, you'll know it's strong, and you won't be ambushed by a poor letter written by someone who perhaps doesn't think that favorably of you. Believe me, this happens all the time and can be the kiss of death when your application is being scored.

4. Know *how* to write it.

How do you get your referrers to allow you to write your own letters of recommendation? Easy, prepare the letters ahead of time, ask them to review them, make any corrections they feel necessary, and that's it. And why would they allow you to write your own letters of recommendation? Think about it; if you know these people well, and they are willing to sign a strong letter of recommendation, you're actually doing them a favor by saving them time. The other benefit of writing the letter yourself, is knowing that it will be submitted on time.

There are three key elements to a good letter of recommendation:

1. Introduction and background of the writer
2. Writer's relationship to the candidate
3. Quantifiable claims rather than generalized statements

EFFECTIVE PHRASES FOR LETTERS OF RECOMMENDATION

The admissions committee will look for your referrer to evaluate you in five specific areas, with strong phrases to support each.

1. MOTIVATION

- ► Displays high energy and drive
- ► Displays a strong incentive to succeed
- ► Strives for excellence at every opportunity
- ► Displays highly motivated inner drive
- ► Displays a strong sense of purpose
- ► Displays a sustained commitment
- ► Displays an enthusiastic spirit
- ► Displays energy and enthusiasm
- ► Inspires enthusiasm
- ► Is able to highly motivate others
- ► Welcomes existing challenges
- ► Thrives on challenges
- ► Displays positive energy
- ► Goes beyond what is expected
- ► Views problems as opportunities
- ► Turns past failures into future successes
- ► Looks beyond obstacles
- ► Is persistent in achieving goals
- ► Is results oriented
- ► Maintains self-motivation

2. INTERPERSONAL SKILLS

- ▶ Displays talent, enthusiasm, and commitment
- ▶ Identifies and understands personal values of superiors, subordinates, peers, and others
- ▶ Demonstrates strong interpersonal skills
- ▶ Is able to quickly establish rapport
- ▶ Builds trust and rapport
- ▶ Excels in trust building
- ▶ Promotes relationships of trust and respect
- ▶ Develops mutual support
- ▶ Develops positive working relationships
- ▶ Promotes harmony among associates

3. MATURITY

- ▶ Displays a high degree of emotional maturity
- ▶ Excels in separating emotion from rationality
- ▶ Copes constructively with emotions
- ▶ Avoids overreacting
- ▶ Maintains strong self-control

4. ABILITY TO HANDLE STRESS

- ▶ Makes strong mental preparations for stressful situations
- ▶ Is very successful in encouraging acceptance of new methods, procedures, and other changes
- ▶ Is able to capably adjust to ever-changing work environments
- ▶ Provides support to employees coping with change
- ▶ Adjusts promptly and calmly to change
- ▶ Is able to cope with pressure and maintain composure
- ▶ Performs well under pressure

5. ACADEMIC PERFORMANCE

- ▶ Ranks in top 10 percent of students I've taught
- ▶ Performs consistently above average
- ▶ Is always prepared for class and exams
- ▶ Is an exceptional student

- ▸ Displays strong analytical qualities
- ▸ Demonstrates a strong ability to analyze problems
- ▸ Is very methodical in solving problems
- ▸ Excels in analyzing and adjusting work procedures for maximum efficiency
- ▸ Excels in analytical thinking

You are now armed with positive phrases that you can include in an effective letter of recommendation. Of course, these phrases must be supported by facts. If your referrer asks you to provide bullet points in order to help him or her write your letter, these are great phrases to include, backed up with facts.

Exercise: Choose three candidates to write your letters of recommendation

List three candidates who would provide a strong and positive letter of recommendation in support of your application:

1. _____

2. _____

3. _____

Now list three backup candidates in case one or more of the above are not available or willing to provide a strong and positive LOR:

1. _____

2. _____

3. _____

Be sure to allow plenty of time to discuss the importance of the LOR with your candidates and ask in plenty of time to meet the CASPA deadline.

CHAPTER 7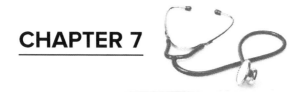

The Essay

If you were to poll a hundred PA school admissions committee members, 99 percent of them would probably agree that the essay (personal statement) is the most important part of the application process. By the time you're ready to submit your application, your grades, test scores, and medical experience are already set in stone, so the essay is your best chance to personalize your application. It's a way for you to make an emotional connection on paper, giving the reader of your essay a strong desire to meet you.

Think about it: admissions committee members may review ten to twenty applications per day. If the essay is "vanilla," it probably won't have much of an impact on the reader. The goal is to write such a compelling essay that the reader can't wait to meet you in person. The essay can even be a tool to explain or make up for less than average grades, test scores, or medical experience.

The purpose of the PA school essay is to really *sell yourself* to the reader. Why should the reader buy your story? Why are you a better applicant than the one whose application was just reviewed?

This chapter provides you with an overview of strategies that will prepare you to write. I offer you commonsense advice that is important in getting you on the right track when writing your PA school essay.

GENERAL TIPS FOR WRITING SUCCESSFUL ESSAYS

1. Express motivation.
2. Demonstrate effective communication skills.
3. Discuss your soft skills.
4. Be real.
5. Be personal.
6. Use details.
7. Tell a story.
8. Be honest.

During that first quick look at your file (transcripts, science and nonscience GPAs, MCAT scores, application, recommendations, and personal statement), every admissions committee seeks essentially the same elements:

- ▸ Proven ability to succeed
- ▸ Clear intellectual ability, analytical and critical thinking skills
- ▸ Evidence that this person has the potential to make not just a good PA student but a good PA

But what they look for when they hone in on your essay is much more than this. We will discuss in detail the things that most admissions committee members list as the most important.

Express Motivation

Your application to PA school is a reflection of your desire to ultimately be a PA. The admissions committee will look to your essay to see that you've answered the obvious but not so simple question—*Why?* You must be able to explain your motivation for attending PA school and for wanting to become a PA.

As an admissions committee member, I looked for a sustained understanding of why candidates wanted to practice medicine, how they had tested their interest, and how they had prepared for PA school.

Touch on your passion to pursue medicine. For many, medicine is akin to a calling, and it is compelling for the evaluators to sense that they are hearing and responding to the same motivation.

I will offer lots of advice in the upcoming pages, and it will be peppered with plenty of dos and don'ts. In the midst of all of this, whatever you do, keep your focus on the ultimate goal of the essay: you must convince the admissions committee that you deserve a seat in their PA program. Everything I tell you should be used as a means to this end, so step back from the details regularly to remind yourself of the big picture.

The essay is the venue for the candidate to make the argument as to why he or she, among all the highly qualified candidates, should be invited for an interview, admitted to PA school, and achieve the ultimate goal of becoming a practicing PA.

Exercise: Expressing emotion in the essay

These are not the easiest questions to answer. However, if you take the time to complete this exercise to the best of your ability, you will be able to write a much more effective essay. You will also discover your strengths and weaknesses as a physician assistant school applicant and identify where you need to improve. The answers to these questions will not only help you write a much more effective essay, they will serve you just as well at the interview.

Answer the following questions.

1. Given your background, how will you demonstrate that you have a proven ability to succeed?

_____

_____

_____

_____

_____

_____

_____

_____

_____

2. How will you discuss the fact that you have clear intellectual ability, as well as analytical and critical thinking skills?

_____

_____

_____

_____

_____

_____

_____

_____

_____

3. What evidence can you produce to show that you would be not only a good PA school student but also a good PA?

_____

_____

_____

_____

_____

_____

_____

_____

4. Why do you want to practice medicine?

_____

_____

_____

_____

_____

_____

_____

_____

5. How have you tested the fact that you want to practice medicine?

_____

_____

_____

_____

_____

_____

_____

_____

6. What have you done to prepare for PA school?

_____

_____

_____

_____

_____

_____

_____

_____

_____

_____

Demonstrate Effective Communication Skills

In the essay, provide a clear sense that you understand and can communicate well the reasons you are a compelling candidate.

Keep in mind that at this level, good writing skills are not sought—they are expected. The committee will look to the essay to ensure strong English language skills, especially if you did some or all of your prerequisite course work in another country. So while a beautifully written essay alone isn't going to get you into PA school, a poorly written one could keep you out of it.

Exercise: How will you demonstrate that you are a compelling candidate for PA school?

Answer to the best of your ability.

_____

_____

_____

_____

_____

_____

_____

_____

_____

_____

_____

_____

_____

_____

_____

_____

_____

_____

Beyond showcasing your writing abilities and demonstrating your motivation, what else can the essay do for you? Let's take a look at what else the committee hopes to find when they read your essay.

Discuss Your Soft Skills

Let the rest of your application—not the personal statement—speak for your hard skills and achievements (i.e., your academic excellence, your fantastic GRE scores, your class rank). What admissions committees seek in the essay are some specific soft skills such as sincerity, maturity, empathy, compassion, depth, and motivation. These qualities were rated especially high in the medical community—more so than for any other graduate-level program studied. Here are some examples to consider:

- _Motivation_
- _Commitment_
- _Sincerity_
- _Honesty_
- _Maturity_
- _Uniqueness_
- _Interest_
- _Sensitivity_

- _Compassion_
- _Empathy_
- _Communication skills_
- _Humanitarian beliefs_
- _Enthusiasm_
- _Creativity_
- _Diversity_

These qualities are not quantifiable and therefore not easily demonstrated.

Many of the essays I have edited and reviewed demonstrate in one way or another that the writers have the soft skills necessary to be good PAs. A few of them even came right out and said it:

"Motivation, independence, maturity, precisely those qualities my experiences in eastern Europe instilled, will be essential to a fruitful career."

But when qualities are mentioned as directly as this, applicants must be careful to support the claims with clear evidence as gathered from personal experience. More often, they just let their achievements and experiences speak for themselves, and the qualities that they demonstrate are inferred.

Exercise: What soft skills will you include in your essay?

List five of the qualities listed on the previous page that you will be able to support in your personal statement.

1. _____

2. _____

3. _____

4. _____

5. _____

How will you support quality #1?

_____

_____

_____

_____

_____

How will you support quality #2?

_____

_____

_____

_____

_____

How will you support quality #3?

_____

_____

_____

_____

_____

How will you support quality #4?

_____

_____

_____

_____

_____

How will you support quality #5?

_____

_____

_____

_____

_____

Be Real

More than any specific skill or characteristic, what admissions committee members seek in the personal statement is a real, live human being.

The members of a PA school admissions committee are responsible for choosing the next generation of physician assistants. These are the people who will be healing our children, curing our parents, and literally saving lives. Put in that perspective, the responsibility the readers feel is enormous. For this reason, they are going to choose to accept someone they feel they know, trust, and like.

In light of this fact, it might not surprise you that when I asked admissions officers and PA students for their top piece of advice regarding the essay, I received the same response almost every time. Although it was expressed in many different ways (be honest, be sincere, be unique, be personal, etc.), it all came down to the same point: be yourself!

My number one piece of advice is to be yourself when you write the essay. The medical profession is a lifetime commitment; let them truly know what drives you toward it!

Unfortunately, achieving this level of communication in writing does not come naturally to everyone. But that does not mean it cannot be learned. Once you understand the basic factors that go into personable writing, you will see that it is not as hard as it seems.

Part of what can make this kind of writing seem so difficult is that it is very hard to gauge the image you are projecting through your writing. Even if you have followed every tip in this book, it is a good idea to have someone objective—preferably someone who doesn't already know you well—read your essay when you have finished. Ask if he or she got a sense of the kind of person you are or was able to picture you while reading. How close is your reader's description to the one you were trying to present? Then ask if the person your reader pictured is someone that he or she would choose to be treated by in a life-or-death situation!

Exercise: *List three people you will have read your essay and provide feedback*

1. _____

2. _____

3. _____

Be Personal

The only way to let the admissions committee see you as an individual is to make your essay personal. When you do this, your essay will automatically be more interesting and engaging, helping it stand out from the hundreds of others the committee will be reviewing that week.

After personally reading thousands of essays, I would advise a couple of key things. First, make it personal. The most boring, dry essays are those that go on about how the applicant *loves science* and *loves working with people* and *wants to serve humanity* but provide few personal details that give a sense of what the applicant is like.

Personalize your essay as much as possible; generic essays are not only boring to read, they're a waste of time because they don't reveal anything about the applicant that helps the reader get to know him or her better.

But what does it mean to make your essay personal? It means that you drop the formalities and write about something that is truly meaningful to you. It means that you include a story or anecdote taken from your life, using lots of details and colorful imagery to give it vitality. And it means, above all, being completely honest.

My database contains many examples of essays that get personal. The following example is one of them. The writer begins by recollecting her experience with anorexia and her admiration of the PA who saved her life. But it is more than this story that makes her essay real—it is the way that she describes her experiences. She uses a real, personal tone throughout the essay; for example, read how she describes herself volunteering at an AIDS clinic:

"I am constantly reminded of how much I have to learn. I look at a baby and notice its cute, pudgy toes. Mary V. [PA-C] plays with it while conversing with its mother, and in less than a minute has noted its responsiveness, strength, and attachment to its parent, and checked its reflexes, color, and hydration. Gingerly, I search for the tympanic membrane in the ears of a cooperative child and touch an infant's warm, soft belly, willing my hands to have a measure of Mary V.'s competence."

It is this writer's admission that she doesn't yet know everything she needs to know, coupled with the picture she paints of herself noticing a baby's "cute, pudgy toes" and "gingerly" searching in "the ears of a cooperative child" and touching "an infant's warm, soft belly" that sets her essay apart. It is hard not to get a feel of the individual who has painted this vivid portrayal using such personal details.

This writer did not rely on her tale of anorexia to make her essay personal. As one admissions officer put it, "A personal epiphany, tragedy, life change, or earth-shattering event is not essential to a strong essay."

This cannot be stressed enough. Personal does not have to mean heavy or emotional or even inspiring. It is a small minority of students who will truly have had a life-changing event to write about. Perhaps an applicant spent time living abroad or experienced death or disease from close proximity. But this is the exception, not the rule.

In fact, students who rely too heavily on weighty experiences often do themselves a disservice. They often don't think about what has really touched them or interests them because they are preoccupied with the topic they think will impress the committee. They write about their grandfather's death because they think that only death (or the emotional equivalent) is significant enough to make them seem deep and mature. But what often happens is that they rely on the experience itself to speak for them and never explain what it meant to them or give a solid example of how it changed them. In other words, they don't make it personal.

Exercise: *List three examples of how you will personalize your essay*

1. _____

2. _____

3. _____

Use Details

To make your essay personal, learn from the example above and use details. Show, don't tell, who you are by backing your claims with real past experiences.

Essays only really help you if they are unique and enable the interviewer to get a sense of who you are based on examples, scenarios, and ideas, rather than lists of what you've done. The readers want to find out *who you are*, not what you have done, although the two are obviously interrelated. Additionally, everything you've "done" is already in the CASPA application.

The key words are *examples*, *scenarios*, and *ideas*. Using detail means getting specific. Each and every point you make needs to be backed up by specific instances taken from your experience. It is these details that make your story special, unique, and interesting.

Look at a excerpt of sentences used in one writer's essay. The writer describes herself gently rocking her first patient:

"… taking care not to disturb the jumbled array of tubes that overwhelmed his tiny body." She says she has "worked with everything from paper-mache to popsicle sticks" and that the children in her ward talk about "Nintendo or the latest Disney movie."

This level of detail is the difference between a personal, interesting story and a yawn-inducing account that could be attributed to any of a thousand applicants.

Exercise: List examples, scenarios, and ideas that you will use in your essay

Write a detailed example of what you may include in your essay.

_____

_____

_____

_____

_____

Brainstorm and document a few scenarios that would create interest in your essay.

1. _____

_____

_____

_____

2. _____

_____

_____

_____

3. _____

_____

_____

_____

What vision do you have for your future as a PA?

_____

_____

_____

_____

_____

Tell a Story

Stories always make for more interesting reading, and they usually convey something more personal than blanket statements like "I want to help people."

Incorporating a story into your essay can be a great way to make it interesting and enjoyable. The safest and most common method of integrating a story into an essay is to tell the story first, then step back into the role of narrator and explain why you presented it and what lessons you learned. This method forces you to begin with the action, which is a surefire way to get the readers' attention and keep them reading.

Many of the essay examples in my database make effective use of storytelling. One begins with a storm at sea, one with a tale of stage fright before a theater performance, and one with a newspaper clipping about the writer as a child. Another writer takes an even more creative approach to the story method by incorporating the story of a prehistoric woman whose bones he has analyzed. What all these writers understood is that a story is best used to draw the reader in. It should always relate back to the motivation to attend PA school or the ability to succeed once admitted.

Exercise: Describe your most memorable patient

This exercise will help you document a very personal, believable, and credible story. Be sure to use the patient's first name to make the story more personal. Describe what you learned from that patient or what the patient taught you about medicine or yourself. You can use this scenario as a key part of your essay.

_____

_____

_____

_____

_____

_____

_____

_____

_____

_____

_____

_____

_____

_____

_____

_____

_____

_____

Be Honest

This last point comes with no caveats and should be upheld without exception. Nothing could be simpler, more straightforward, or more crucial than this: be honest, forthright, and sincere.

Admissions officers have zero tolerance for hype. If you try to be something that you're not, it will be transparent to the committee. You will come off as immature at best and unethical at worst. If you say that one of your favorite hobbies is playing chess, then you'd better have a favorite opening move. When the admissions committee members read your essay the day of the interview, one of them might be an expert player and want to swap techniques!

As a former PA admissions committee member, I can say that it is so important to be honest. The students are asked many times about their personal statements when interviewing, and it's painfully obvious when they exaggerate or are overly dramatic when recounting their experiences.

When you are honest about your motivations and goals, you will come across as more personable and real. One essayist, for example, begins,

> *"When I entered Quinnipiac University in 2004, I was amazed by the large number of students already labeled as 'pre-physician assistant.' I wondered how those students were able to decide with such certainty that they wanted to study medicine, and I imagined that they all must have known from a very early age that they would one day be great PAs. I had no such inklings, and if asked as a child what I wanted to be when I grew up, I would have said that I wanted to be an Olympic skier or soccer player."*

Because of the plethora of essays that begin with "I've wanted to be a physician assistant for as long as I can remember," this writer's honest approach must have been refreshing and memorable for readers.

Exercise: Document at least one vignette that you may be able to use in your essay

_____

_____

_____

_____

_____

_____

_____

_____

_____

If you want your application to stand out from the crowd, you must make an emotional connection on paper. In order to do this, follow these simple rules:

1. Use vignettes (small, illustrative sketches) to tell a story and keep your reader interested.
2. Avoid spelling errors. One spelling error can doom your entire application. Paying strict attention to detail is a key attribute of health care professionals.
3. Limit the use of the word "I;" instead, use "we," "us," and "our" to show that you are not self-centered and that you are a team player. (Note, one PA program director instructs attendees at the open house, "If you have more than five 'I's in your essay, do it over!")
4. Answer the question that is being asked of you.
5. Don't rely on your spell checker. A great tip is to read your essay backward, from the last word to the first word, and spelling and grammatical errors will pop out at you.

The essay can be the great equalizer. I've personally reviewed hundreds of applications where the candidate had an excellent GPA, test scores, and medical experience but blew it on the essay. Put a great deal of thought and preparation into your essay so that the reader has a strong desire to meet you (and find out more about you) after reading it.

TEN COMMON ERRORS SPELL CHECK WON'T CATCH

When I served on the PA school admissions committee at Yale, my personal pet peeve was spelling errors on the essay. Most committee members agree; just one spelling or grammatical error on the essay can be catastrophic. The logic is, if you miss a spelling or grammatical error on your application, will you miss a critical lab value or diagnosis on a patient?

With only a 5 percent chance of acceptance for the most competitive programs, you need to avoid spelling or grammatical errors at all costs. Here are ten common errors spell check won't catch:

- **"Its" versus "It's"** (and all other contractions): Mixing these two up is the most common error in the English language. Learn the difference.

- **"Sales" versus "Sails"**

- **"Affect" versus "Effect:"** There is a lot of confusion about this one, but here's the rule: "affect" is usually a verb, and "effect" is usually a noun.

- **"Would have,"** *not* **"Would of:"** "Would of" is never correct and may make you appear as if you are not well-read.

- **"Through" versus "Threw:"** He threw the ball through the window. "Threw" is a verb, and "through" is a preposition. And speaking of "through," be careful to make sure you don't actually mean "thorough" or vice versa. The slight variation in spelling will not be picked up by a computer, but writing, "I am through," when you mean, "I am thorough," is quite ironic, don't you think?

- **"Then" versus "Than:"** Six is more than five; after five then comes six. "Than" refers to comparison, while "then" refers to a subsequent event.

- **"Supposed to,"** *not* **"Suppose to:"** "Suppose" is a verb meaning to think or to ponder. The correct way to express a duty is to write, "I was supposed to . . ."

- **"Wonder" versus "Wander"**

- **"Their" versus "There" versus "They're:"** "Their" is possessive, "there" refers to distance, and "they're" is a contraction of "they are."

- **"Farther" versus "Further"**: While both words refer to distance, grammarians distinguish "farther" as physical distance and "further" as metaphorical distance. You can dive *further* into a project, for instance, or you can dive *farther* into the ocean.

THINKING STRATEGICALLY

Understanding the Writing Process

One common misunderstanding about good writing is that it is the result of moments of inspiration. While these moments can be helpful, good writing is not the result of inspiration—rather, it is the result of hard work and numerous rewrites. So before you start, know that an effective essay will take some time.

Further, the best writing doesn't just "happen" when you sit down. Good writing requires preparation and then multiple drafts. Be prepared to work through several drafts and sit through many writing sessions.

Preparation for good writing also requires forethought. Think about what you want to say, as well as how you want to say it; let an idea roll around in your mind a bit, and then try committing it to paper. Being strategic about writing can improve your chances of creating a winning essay.

Where to Write

Some people need a quiet room with a desk. Others prefer a noisy coffee shop. According to a *Chicago Tribune* article entitled "Where Writers Write," many famous writers have very specific requirements about their inspirational places to put pen to paper. Oscar Hijuelos (*The Mambo Kings Play Songs of Love*) needs a quiet, private space, preferably with a view. Jodi Picoult (author of numerous novels) writes in her attic office. Tayari Jones (*Silver Sparrow*) writes in the spare bedroom of her apartment. And Wally Lamb (*She's Come Undone* and many others) prefers his finished basement for writing.

While you aren't writing a novel, you still need to consider where you do your best thinking and writing and try to work in that setting each and every time you write. Your mind will automatically shift into writing mode if you follow a routine related to where and when you write. While this may seem like an unnecessary step in the writing process, remember that your PA essay has the potential to change the trajectory of your life. Spending a bit of time to think about space can be an important part of your process.

When to Write

It is important to think about when you should write. Some people like to write early in the morning, when they feel fresh. Others like to write late at night.

Don't plan to write at a time when your creative brain has shut down (writing is a creative process, after all) or after you have just completed an intense mental task (e.g., a test). Think about when you do your best writing, and plan to work on your essay during that time.

Stimulating the Writing Brain

It's happened to all of us. You sit down with a pen and paper or at your computer and . . . nothing. You don't know how to start, and nothing is coming from your blocked brain. Never fear; even great writers need stimulation at times. Are you someone for whom reading stimulates your desire to write? Or does journaling get your creative juices flowing? Or maybe you find that quiet meditation gets you into the writing mood. Having a writing routine will help you when you begin writing your essay.

Here are some fun exercises to get your mind ready to write:

1. Write down fifty adjectives to describe yourself.
2. Write a paragraph or two about your life five years from now, when you are a successful PA. What do you like about your job? What do you enjoy about being with patients? What do you like about the practice of medicine?
3. Write a fictional story about a PA hero or heroine. What would he or she do? Who are this PA's patients? What do these patients think of your hero or heroine?
4. Talk aloud (to yourself or a friend) about what you want to say in your essay or how you might start it. If you are a very verbal person, this can be a great way to get your writing brain engaged.
5. Write one sentence each about five people you admire and what you admire about them.

These are just a few examples of ways to get warmed up for writing. Just like in physical exercise, warm-ups can be helpful. The Internet is filled with suggestions for writing warm-ups, so if none of these ideas inspire you and you are still not sure how to start, check online.

Scheduling and Deadlines

Remember to also put yourself on a schedule. Create a timeline that includes deadlines for making an outline, completing a first draft, doing revisions, and finally finishing the essay. Put these deadlines into your cell phone calendar as reminders. Allow yourself adequate time for all creative processes, as well as revisions and edits. Often, starting at the end (the deadline) and working backward with your schedule will allow you to see the quantity of time you will need to dedicate to this task.

While deadlines can be hard for some people, they provide the structure for keeping organized. Remember to include in your schedule flexibility for personal and family emergencies, other work deadlines or commitments, computer problems, etc. The last thing you want to be in a position to have to do is miss the CASPA deadline.

Managing Writer's Block

Finally, prepare for writer's block. Even professional writers get stumped at times. If your writing gets stalled, it is probably your brain telling you it is time for a break—so take one.

Do free writing exercises, go for a walk, or get a cup of coffee or tea. In summary, distracting yourself for a minute or ten minutes can give the writing part of your brain enough of a break that it is fresh and ready to start again when you return.

Procrastination

Everyone procrastinates at times, and students have been known to procrastinate more than others. Rather than work, we surf the Internet, clean our closets, use social media, etc. While everyone procrastinates at times, it is estimated that 20 percent of all people are procrastinators. If you are one of those people, there is hope, but you will need to be disciplined.

Here are some tips:

1. Estimate correctly. Some of us procrastinate because we've underestimated how long it takes to do something—and we know it. If you see a trend, adapt. In other words, if tasks usually take two times longer than you expect, schedule a task to take two times longer.
2. Make a list, and set a schedule.
3. Set realistic goals. As I have mentioned and will mention again later in this book, your essay will not be effective if you sit and write it in one session. So be realistic about what you can do.
4. Promise yourself a reward when you complete your tasks.
5. Repeat the mantra: "Just do it now!"

Use a checklist to prepare for writing your essay:

1. I have identified a specific location from which I can do my best writing.
2. I have identified the best time of day for writing.
3. I know several strategies for stimulating my brain to write.
4. I have developed a schedule for completing my application essay.
5. I created deadlines for completion of parts of my essay and proofing and editing.
6. I know what to do to move beyond writer's block.
7. I know what to do when I am procrastinating to move myself to action.

EVOLUTION OF AN ESSAY

When applying to PA school, consider your essay to be your ticket to the interview. A quality essay answers the question as to what motivates you to want to become a PA. The CASPA essay may be the most important piece of medical writing that you do in your entire career. When writing the essay, remember the following:

- Capture the **attention** of the reader right from the beginning. Admissions committee members read hundreds of essays each cycle and become bored with essays that don't capture the attention of the reader instantly.

- Create **interest** in your essay by telling a story or writing vignettes to keep the reader captivated.

- Show **conviction** in your essay by giving plenty of supporting examples of why you are choosing this profession.

- Create a strong **desire** in your essay that will compel the reader to want to learn more about you.

- **Close** the deal by summarizing your essay with a strong finish that will entice the reader to score you high and ask you to come for an interview.

Writing a great essay can be extremely difficult for some applicants. After all, if you fail to connect with the reader on an emotional level, you will probably fail to receive an interview. Use my essay review and editing services (andrewrodican.com) to rest assured that your essay will be compelling, error-free, and ready to cut and paste into your CASPA application.

I've included a sample edit I performed for an applicant. The directions for the essay were clear:

Attach to this application a typewritten narrative of not more than two pages, explaining where you learned of the PA profession, what factors or influences led you to this career choice, and how you expect to fulfill your goals as a physician assistant.

The following original essay was sent to AJR Associates (andrewrodican.com) for review and editing.

All around me is nothing but a wide open field of alfalfa hay. The sweet smell of honeysuckle in the air brings about a feeling of relaxation as I ride on the green John Deere. To the left, the hay has been raked in single file rows, ready to be baled. To my right, is a blanket of hay needing to be raked in a line before it gets too dry from the warm July sun. My father arrives at the field entrance and is unhooking the gate so he can pull his blue Ford tractor and baler through.

Every summer my dad and I each spend about three hundred hours on tractors baling hay for our cattle in preparation for the snowy winter months. This lifestyle is common among the people in my community. I adore my small hometown, and my desire is to return there as a health care provider—another field I love.

Working on a beef farm and making hay have always brought me self-fulfillment. I shadowed a large-animal veterinarian thinking that was the right path for me; but after the veterinarian himself said, "This job is not for you if you want to raise a family because as a large-animal veterinarian, you will be on call all day and night," I decided against this career. I truly enjoy taking care of animals and treating them for their illnesses, but the veterinary route is not for me. Deep within, I knew I had a desire to care for people and this nurturing characteristic of mine brought health care to my attention as a potential career. For a high school project, I shadowed a pharmacist at Wytheville Community Hospital. I thought this would be a prestigious and satisfying career. In fact, I pursued pharmacology until my sophomore year in college; however, I knew there was something missing. Numerous hours at a counter filing prescriptions and assisting the pharmacist at the University of Virginia Outpatient Pharmacy became monotonous quickly.

My best friend called me one day as I was walking to my organic chemistry class. I told her that I was having second thoughts about becoming a pharmacist. When she asked me why, I responded along the lines of, "I need more interaction with people; that connection would keep a job interesting and challenging. I have a passion for providing assistance directly to people." She mentioned med school, but immediately I answered, "Med school is not for me. I do not want to go to school for that long; I do not want to have an enormous amount of debt upon graduation; and mainly, I do not want the liability a doctor is burdened with." She said, "Why not be a Physician Assistant?" That moment was when I first heard of a physician assistant. I was confused as to what a physician assistant did, so I began to do some research. I subscribed to the undergraduate Physician Assistant Club email list at University of Virginia and attended a few meetings. I fell in love with the idea of becoming a Physician Assistant. The speaker at one of the meetings was from a college that had a Physician Assistant Program. He discussed how physician assistants worked autonomously yet collaboratively with physicians. He highlighted versatility and described how

Physician Assistants are in high demand, particularly in rural areas. All of these characteristics of a physician assistant were appealing, and I knew this career was what I wanted. Many discussions with my parents, family members, friends, and professors solidified that this profession was something I wanted to pursue. I contacted a family physician assistant working in my hometown, and she allowed me to shadow her. We discussed the pros and cons of being a physician assistant; and we quickly determined this was a perfect career choice for me. I enjoyed watching her interact with her patients, yet she had the security of knowing she could refer to a physician for aide when a case needed further opinions. My humble, conscientious and ethical personality allows me to be independent, yet willing to consider other recommendations when necessary—essential characteristics that promotes quality health care.

Three months ago, a close friend of mine was diagnosed with Squamous Cell Carcinoma. This diagnosis was a shock to his wife, son and me. He scheduled an appointment for surgery, follow-up radiation, and chemotherapy. My friend, being diagnosed with such an illness and knowing he would have to undergo these treatments, was feeling sincerely scared and worried for his survival. Yet he had trust and faith in all of the health care staff to rid him of his cancer. His wife and son were putting all of their hope in the doctors, nurses, and physician assistants as well. The head of their household, their rock and provider, was put in these medical providers hands. I am passionate about establishing a caring, empathetic and resolute patient-physician and family-physician relationship, founded upon trust, faith and hope. For patients to put their hope and trust in my hands as a practicing physician assistant and to give them and/or their family members quality health care is a goal I long to fulfill; one that would leave me with a satisfying and purposeful feeling each day.

My long-term goal is to become a Physician Assistant, practice in my rural hometown in Southwest Virginia, and build a trusting patient-physician relationship that demands the best health care possible. This dream would give me a life-long feeling of what I experience when riding the John Deere, making sweet-smelling alfalfa hay on a warm, breezy summer's day.

Now read the same essay with edits made to enhance it:

I'm in the middle of an open field of alfalfa hay. The sweet smell of honeysuckle in the air **relaxes me** as I ride on the green John Deere. To **my** left, the hay has been raked in single-file rows, ready to be bailed. To my right is a blanket of hay needing to be raked to the right before **the hot**

July sun dries it out. *My father* **calls to me from** *the field entrance* **as he** *unhook***s** *the gate* **to** *pull his blue Ford tractor and bailer through. There is more to do.*

Corrections to paragraph 1
Deleted: All ... around me is nothing but ... a wide ... brings ... about a feeling of relaxation ... the ... , ... it gets too dry from the warm July sun. arrives ... at ... and is ... ing ... so ... he .Every ... This lifestyle is common among the ... my desire ... can ...

Each *summer my dad and I each spend about three hundred hours on tractors bailing hay for our cattle in preparation for the snowy winter months,* **a common activity for** *people in my community. I adore my small home town, and* **my dream is** *to return there* **to fulfill my other passion—to serve my community** *as a health care provider.*

Corrections to paragraph 2
Deleted: Every ... This lifestyle is common among the ... my desire ... as a health care provider—another field I love

Working on a beef farm **has** *always* **fed my soul**. *I shadowed a large-animal veterinarian, thinking that* **veterinary medicine might be** *the right path for me, but the veterinarian* **cautioned me against the field if I wanted** *to raise a family because* **I would** *be on call day and night.* **Though** *taking care of animals* **appeals to my nurturing spirit, this experience shifted my focus to a deeper interest in taking care of** *people,* **which** *brought health care to my attention as a career.* **While in** *high school, I shadowed a pharmacist at Wytheville Community Hospital,* **thinking pharmacy might** *be a satisfying career. I pursued pharmacology until my sophomore year in college,* **when my experience at the University of Virginia Outpatient Pharmacy showed me that spending all day** *at a counter fil*l*ing prescriptions and* **helping** *the pharmacist* **was simply too** *monotonous* **and isolated for me**.

Corrections to paragraph 3
Deleted: and ... making having brought me self-fulfillment ... was; ... after ... himself said ... "This job is not for you if you want ... as a large animal ... veterinarian, you will ... all, ... " ... I decided against this career ... .I truly enjoy ... and treating them for their illnesses, but the veterinarian route is not for me. Deep within, ... I knew ... I ... had a desire to care for ... and this nurturing characteristic of mine ... potential ... For ... a ... project ... I thought this would prestigious and ... In fact, ... ;however ... I knew there was something missing ... .Numerous hours ... assisting all the University of Virginia Outpatient Pharmacy became ... quickly.

A light bulb went off one day as I was speaking with my *best friend. I* **shared with** *her that I was having second thoughts about* *pharmacy* **and that I craved** *more interaction with people. She* **asked if I had considered going to** *med school, but* **I had a litany of reasons why that was not for me, including the length of time it takes to finally be able to practice, the enormous debt I would accrue, and the liability doctors are burdened with**. *She said, "Why not be a* **p**hysician *assistant?"* **Though I hate to admit it, that was the first time I had even** *heard of* **the role, so I started doing my research**. *I* **explored** *the undergraduate Physician Assistant Club at* **the** *University of Virginia* **and soon** *fell in love with the idea of becoming a* **PA. At one club meeting, a** *speaker from a* **PA** *p*rogram **explained** *how physician assistants work autonomously yet collaboratively with physicians.* **He highlighted the** *versatility* **of the career** *and described how* **PAs** *are in high demand, particularly in rural areas.* **Like a bolt of lightning, it struck me that this was the perfect path for me.** *I* **began shadowing** *a family physician assistant in my hometown,* **who spoke about** *the* **opportunities and challenges** *of being a physician assistant. I* **loved the fact that she had direct patient interaction while being able to** *refer* **questions** *to a physician when she needed further opinions.* **I knew that this balance of independence and collaboration suited my personality to a tee, but it was a personal encounter with health care that cemented my passion for the profession.**

Corrections to paragraph 4

Deleted: M … called me one day as I was walking to my Organic chemistry class … told … becoming a … ist … When she asked me why, I responded along the lines of, "I need … ; that connection would keep a job interesting and challenging … I have the passion for providing assistance directly to people." Mentioned … immediately … I answered, "Med school is not for me. I do not want to go to school for that long. I do not want to have an enormous amount of debt upon graduation; and mainly, I do not want the liability a doctor is burdened with." … P … A … That moment was when I first … a physician assistant … I was confused as to what a physician assistant did, so I began to do some research. Subscribed … to … email list … and attended a few meetings. I … Physician Assistant … … The … at one of the meetings was … college that had a Physician Assistant … P … He discussed … ed … Physician … Assistants … All of these characteristics of a physician assistant were appealing, and I knew … this career was what I wanted. Many discussions with my parents, family members, friends, and professors solidified that this profession was something I wanted to pursue … contacted … working … and she allowed me to shadow her … We discussed … pros and cons … ;and we quickly determined this was a perfect career choice for me … … enjoyed watching … her interact with her patients, yet she had the security of knowing she could … for … aide when a case … My humble , conscientious and ethical personality allows me to be independent, yet willing to consider other recommendations when necessary--essential characteristics that promote

Three months ago, a close friend of mine was diagnosed with squamous cell carcinoma, **a shock to his family and friends.** *He* **was thrown into a blur of** *appointment**s** for surgery, radiation, and chemotherapy.* **Worried about** *his* **potential for** *survival,* **he and his wife and son were left with no choice but to put** *their faith in the health care staff*—**from physicians to PAs to nurses**—*to save his life.* **I saw the difference made by the bedside manner of those caring for him, both positive and negative, and became even more** *passionate about establishing a caring, empathetic, and* **devoted** *patient-physician and family-physician relationship. For patients to put their trust in my hands* **will be a tremendous honor** *that* **will give** *me* **a tremendous sense of purpose** *each day.*

Corrections to paragraph 5

Deleted: ... This diagnosis was a shock to his wife, son and me ... .scheduled ... an ... follow-up ... My friend, being diagnosed with such an illness and knowing he would have to undergo these treatments, was ... feeling sincerely scared and worried for ... . Yet he had trust and ... all of ... rid ... him of his cancer ... His wife and son were putting all their hope in the doctors, nurses, and physician assistants as well ... .The head of their household, their rock and provider, was put in these medical providers hands. I am ... ... resolute ... , founded upon trust, faith and hope ... hope and ... as a practicing physician assistant and to give them and/or their ... would ... leave ... with ... satisfying and purposeful

My goal is to **practice** **as** *a* **p**hysician **a**ssistant in my rural hometown in Southwest Virginia, build**ing** trusting patient-physician relationship**s** **and impacting the overall health of my community. As I drive by the lines of fields on my way to work as a PA, the sweet scent of alfalfa and honeysuckle will reassure me that I am right where I am supposed to be.**

Corrections to paragraph 6

Deleted: long ... -term ... become ... P ... A ... , practice ... and ... a ... that ... demands the best health care ... This dream would give me

Compare the version above with the final draft of this essay:

I'm in the middle of an open field of alfalfa hay. The sweet smell of honeysuckle in the air relaxes me as I ride on the green John Deere. To my left, the hay has been raked in single-file rows, ready to be baled. To my right is a blanket of hay needing to be raked in a line before the hot July sun dries it out. My father calls to me from the field entrance as he unhooks the gate to pull his blue Ford tractor and baler through. There is more to do.

Each summer my dad and I each spend about three hundred hours on tractors baling hay for our cattle in preparation for the snowy winter months, a common activity for people in my community. I adore my small hometown, and my dream is to return there to fulfill my other passion—to serve my community as a health care provider.

Working on a beef farm has always fed my soul. I shadowed a large-animal veterinarian, thinking that veterinary medicine might be the right path for me, but the veterinarian cautioned me against the field if I wanted to raise a family because I would be on call day and night. Though taking care of animals appeals to my nurturing spirit, this experience shifted my focus to a deeper interest in taking care of people, which brought health care to my attention as a career. While in high school, I shadowed a pharmacist at Wytheville Community Hospital, thinking pharmacy might be a satisfying career. I pursued pharmacology until my sophomore year in college, when my experience at the University of Virginia Outpatient Pharmacy showed me that spending all day at a counter filling prescriptions and helping the pharmacist was simply too monotonous and isolated for me.

A light bulb went off one day as I was speaking with my best friend. I shared with her that I was having second thoughts about pharmacy and that I craved more interaction with people. She asked if I had considered going to med school, but I had a litany of reasons why that was not for me, including the length of time it takes to finally be able to practice, the enormous debt I would accrue, and the liability doctors are burdened with. She said, "Why not be a physician assistant?" Though I hate to admit it, which was the first time I had even heard of the role, so I started doing my research. I explored the undergraduate Physician Assistant Club at the University of Virginia and soon fell in love with the idea of becoming a PA. At one club meeting, a speaker from a PA program explained how physician assistants work autonomously yet collaboratively with physicians. He highlighted the versatility of the career and described how PAs are in high demand, particularly in rural areas. Like a bolt of lightning, it struck me that this was the perfect path for me. I began shadowing a family physician assistant in my hometown, who spoke about the opportunities and challenges of being a physician assistant. I loved the fact that she had direct patient interaction while being able to refer questions to a physician when she needed further opinions. I knew that this balance of independence and collaboration suited my personality to a tee, but it was a personal encounter with health care that cemented my passion for the profession.

Three months ago, a close friend of mine was diagnosed with squamous cell carcinoma, a shock to his family and friends. He was thrown into a blur of appointments for surgery, radiation, and chemotherapy. Worried about his potential for survival, he and his wife and son were left with no choice but to put their faith in the health care staff—from physicians to PAs to nurses—to save his life. I saw the difference made by the bedside manner of those caring for him, both positive and negative, and became even more passionate about establishing a caring, empathetic, and devoted patient-physician and family-physician relationship. For patients to put their trust in my hands will be a tremendous honor that will give me a tremendous sense of purpose each day.

My goal is to practice as a physician assistant in my rural hometown in Southwest Virginia, building trusting patient-physician relationships and impacting the overall health of my community. As I drive by the lines of fields on my way to work as a PA, the sweet scent of alfalfa and honeysuckle will reassure me that I am right where I am supposed to be.

Here are four more sample essays that worked for others:

Sample Essay 1

My fingertips brushed the ruffled edge of the pink handmade card that was pinned on the wall at Edwards Lifesciences. It was my first day of work, and I was still taking in my surroundings. Although there was quite a buzz of busy employees rushing through the hallway, rattling off complex scientific terminology, my focus was not broken. Amid the hundreds of cards I read walking down the hall, one in particular grabbed my attention; it was written by a child who could not have been more than five years old. In squiggly, childish handwriting were the simple words, "Thank you for saving my life, Dr. Laks."

It was like looking fifteen years back in time, recalling the earliest memory of a story my parents have often told me. My feeding habits as a newborn were unlike those of normal babies. I was consuming milk in scant cubic centimeters instead of ounces. As weeks went by, my weight dropped rapidly. I was taken to many doctors who scoffed at my case, dismissing it as a minor thyroid or digestive disorder. Desperately, my parents rushed me to UCLA Medical Center, where a young female intern knelt down beside me, put her ear to my heart, and noted an irregular beat. Tests later confirmed that I had a congenital heart defect, and I would need surgery soon if I were to survive. At a mere five weeks old, I had emergency open-heart surgery, performed by Dr. Hillel Laks. He patched a dime-sized hole, enormous compared to my little heart. Unwittingly, by way of his expertise and care, Dr. Laks had set my life on a new course.

My parents vividly described the events after the surgery when I was in the ICU, recovering, with multiple tubes coursing through my body. My life hung in the balance, and I live with this story as a constant reminder of life's fragility, acknowledging that I was graciously given a second chance. I believe that growing up with the understanding of my experience has positively shaped my life. These early, deeply buried memories have empowered my commitment and have compelled me to work in medicine so that I can help improve the quality of life for the people I have a chance to serve.

My passion to aid others and provide them with professional yet personal care deepened after a recent poignant experience working in a neurological clinic. It was an ordinary afternoon. I remember waiting for the next patient in a clinic room when an elderly man shuffled through the door, leaning on a cane in his left hand. He entered with a calm but sullen disposition, looked up, and greeted me with a nod. I helped him to a nearby chair and waited for him to begin his story. He had been diagnosed with dementia and was living with a caretaker. His wife had passed away, as had many of his friends. Depressed from having suffered through such isolation, he had lost his vitality and vigor. As he spoke, he stared blankly into the distance, with lifeless marbles for eyes that yearned for a connection. I pulled my chair closer and gently patted his hand. He turned and greeted me with a warm, crooked smile. The smile alone revealed that simply by way of a heartfelt touch, I, as a caregiver, could momentarily free him from his loneliness and ease his suffering. This chance to connect with and provide relief to those in need compels me to meet the medical and emotional needs of others.

Much as my life did at five weeks old, the life of this man hangs tenuously on a precipice, wrought with uncertainty about the future. I learned from talking to this man that treatments may not always be available, but as a physician assistant, I can still offer my patients a gentle touch and the genuine compassion they desire. He has taught me that life, even at its end, warrants humanity.

I pass by the handmade card at Edwards Lifesciences daily, and each time, I am reminded of my life's story. It is a memory that I will always carry with me, for it has spurred within me the desire to give back and to help others. I am endeared to this cause, and it is my personal mission of gratitude to give hope and to provide comfort. It is my way of saying thank you.

Sample Essay 2

At five, I wanted to be a doctor. At forty-nine, my motivation and desire to become a physician assistant is not only historical in nature but deeply rooted. My career, family, personal journey, and spirituality have entwined and culminated into a genuine calling demanding a leap of faith and considerable personal sacrifice.

Desiring to be a physician has always been a part of me. In adolescence, I knew I was designed for the helping professions. My passion was to go to medical school, but I was too immature to make that commitment. Alternatively, I earned a bachelor's degree in psychology, and my hopeful and optimistic step into health care began. As I asserted my duties in psychological services, my quieted longing to become a doctor lingered.

My first work in mental health involved social work, case management, and counseling services with different populations inside a medically based model of services. During those years, my knowledge grew rapidly. I was privileged to work beside outstanding professionals, including doctors and nurses. Successfully managing a family and a full-time career, I earned a master's degree in psychology. I continued to develop clinically, but also I evolved personally to develop an even deeper desire to help others. My experiences broadened to include working in a private psychiatric hospital, among many other opportunities. My keen interest in health and medicine only grew, coinciding with my confidence, expertise, and personal satisfaction. Even in those years, I felt I was being drawn toward something.

The love of my family, my financial responsibilities, and a sudden loss of employment diverted me from mental health and led me into skilled nursing. I was offered the social-services director position in a large, fast-paced skilled-nursing facility. This was not only a managerial position, but it immersed me clinically into the function of its interdisciplinary care team over my fourteen-year tenure. It was partly a dream come true. Not only did I find myself in a position of considerable responsibility, with supervisory and leadership roles, but I was living and learning in the vast expanse of medicine.

Those rigorous days proved to be a continuous training ground. My typical workday walked me through an unpredictable variety of teachable moments. I thrived in it. From the moment I stepped upon "the floor," I was integrally involved with communicating, planning, and treating patients with an array of professionals, including physicians; physician assistants; nurse practitioners; psychiatrists; psychologists;

nurses; certified nursing assistants; dietitians; physical, occupational and speech therapists; even clergy.

Furthermore, hospital engagement was a part of it all. I was routinely discerning medical records, history, and physicals; medication administration records; treatment administration records; and lab work while incorporating this information into my daily responsibilities for our patients.

While working and communicating with patients (and their families), I served real people struggling with real disease, acute injury, and disorienting trauma within this subacute setting.

I was happy! I was fully involved in healing and intimately helping vulnerable people of all walks of life. I was a team member engaged in the practice of medicine. This rekindled the realization that I still had a deep desire to become a medical professional engaged in a practice beyond what I was currently doing. I also came to see and believe that I was capable of such service. I decided that my time had passed to become a physician, but my dream of practicing and serving as a physician assistant was born. I knew that if I were given the chance, I would succeed.

Injury brought me new perspective about the role of the PA. I perforated my esophagus with food, and emergency surgery ensued. I experienced two separate thoracotomies, two weeks thrust into intensive care, one month's infirmity, and the most competent medical care any person could ever receive. Unimaginable pain was managed, and I fully recovered. I decided if there were a will and a way, I would attempt to gain entry into a program. Such would enable me to become a physician assistant and perhaps participate in the level of care and healing that I had received. I found the will.

Before this decision, family members and colleagues encouraged me to apply, offering forceful votes of confidence. Through my prayer life, it has become abundantly clear that I am called to apply and hopefully serve as a physician assistant. With the support of my wife and family, I vacated my career to pursue prerequisite courses needed to apply and ultimately pursue this goal. The solid achievements in every class over that year have further reinforced my desire and have given me confidence that I can successfully complete a physician assistant program.

Moving forward, I hope for the open doors to realize an abiding dream and obey my calling to serve.

Sample Essay 3

"A PA helped save my daughter's life," exclaimed my coworker Christy. She detailed how the persistence and advocacy of a PA at the ER had been instrumental in diagnosing her daughter with Kawasaki syndrome. As she spoke, I was struck—yet again—by the dedication of this PA, not unlike that of the many other PAs I had contacted in prior months. Though I had been exploring the profession for some time already, it was this defining moment that truly cemented my desire to become a PA.

I grew up outside Bombay, India, and my late grandfather had been our town's first doctor; I grew up hearing stories of his love for people and medicine. My grandmother—who suffered a stroke and diabetes—let me "help" her take insulin shots and medication. Though I was young, these experiences left a strong impression; it was during this time my love of service and health care was born.

Growing up in India was a wonderful experience. I learned to interact and live with people of diverse perspectives, cultures, languages, and religions. In March 1993, due to ongoing religious rifts, a string of bombs was set off in downtown Bombay. My father's office building was a target; he was trapped for hours before being rescued. Though he suffered only minor injuries, my family was shaken to its core; we immigrated to Canada shortly thereafter.

In Canada, my father was unable to find a job and succumbed to depression and alcoholism. I started working at fifteen, to help support my mother and younger brother. Though far from ideal, this situation instilled in me excellent time-management skills and a determination to excel. I learned to balance paid work with strong academics and community service. This included volunteer positions at an animal shelter, a sexual- and domestic-violence hotline, a local hospital, an opera house, and with local environmental groups. Working at the crisis hotline and at the hospital, I realized my true desire was to serve people through health care—though I was still unsure of the route I would take.

When accepted to the University of Toronto, I made the difficult decision to continue living at home and supporting my family. Since my decision made me ineligible to receive financial aid, I took on a second job to fund my education. This was a crippling period in my life: emotionally, physically, financially, and academically. Despite a strong desire to excel, and an inherent love of learning, I simply did not have the time or the means to demonstrate my academic ability. Coping with my father's disease—and his increasing verbal and physical outbursts—eroded our family finances and all sense of stability. A heavy work schedule, combined with the increased financial burden of education and a competitive academic environment, meant I could not perform at a level that reflected my true academic abilities. Though dropping out of school would have alleviated much stress, I persisted, determined to graduate in good standing, in my chosen field. Though it was the most challenging time of my life, it taught me maturity, adaptability, and most of all, perseverance. I graduated in good standing in 2006 and moved to Texas shortly after.

In 2007 I began work at Cogenics, as part of a team that provided molecular biology services to a wide range of clients. The technical and logistical challenges of the job were enjoyable, as was the opportunity to expand on knowledge acquired in university. In 2009, I moved to Biotics Research Corporation (BRC), a respected nutraceutical company that manufactured over one hundred unique dietary supplements. Working at BRC was a tremendous growing experience. As the only quality assurance (QA) coordinator, I supervised a team of eight QA associates, as well as acted as a liaison between the board of directors and company-wide QA activity. In this fast-paced environment, I learned crisis management, how to identify and solve unique problems, and most of all, how to effectively work in high-stress situations while maintaining my composure and the integrity of my role. The health-related aspects of this job strongly rekindled my desire to work in health care; I knew without doubt that a future profession based on a medical model of education was my goal.

Shortly after I began work at BRC in 2009, my husband was treated for an eye injury by a PA at our local ER. I was impressed with her depth of knowledge, calm demeanor, and the ease with which she worked alongside the doctor to treat my husband. She was happy to tell me about her journey into the PA profession; that very night began my quest into understanding the profession more fully. I joined the AAPA and contacted as many PAs as possible. In the many phone and e-mail conversations that ensued, two similarities stood out: all loved their chosen profession and the team-oriented nature of their jobs. Both of these were traits I strongly valued in any future profession. In shadowing five PAs, I was amazed at the range and complexity of specialties they practice in—from the ICU to cardiovascular surgery—and also at the unique relationship that exists between each PA and supervising physician. It was also during this time I met Christy and experienced the defining moment that led to this application.

I quit my job in June 2010 and returned to school full-time; I wanted to prove my academic capability and become a more competitive PA candidate. Since then I have completed forty-two hours in PA prerequisites with a 4.0 GPA. I also volunteer in the community as an adult English as a second language (ESL) teacher and at Houston Hospice and most recently at Omega House.

As an adult ESL teacher in an underserved community, I develop curricula and teach adults to speak and write English. All of my students are immigrants who—as I once did—cope with various levels of cultural isolation. Being able to empathize with their situation has helped me not only be a teacher, but a life coach and cheerleader of sorts. I am proud to say that with my help, many have dramatically improved their language skills; some have even gone on to find jobs or complete their GEDs—goals they never thought possible.

At Houston Hospice, I have the honor and privilege of interacting with patients in the final chapter of their lives. Learning to deal with death in medicine was a challenge. Here, I learned that being a good caregiver means more than administering treatments—it means offering empathy and comfort as well. It saddens me that PAs are still unable to practice in this area of medicine; if given the opportunity, I hope to one day be part of the growing PA movement that is trying this.

While at Houston Hospice, a lead nurse recommended I volunteer at Omega House, where she had previously been director of nursing. Omega House is a residential hospice for people in the late stages of HIV/AIDS; volunteers contribute almost 70 percent of patient care. Here, I have had the opportunity to serve patients in many ways: by socializing and interacting with them; cooking meals, changing clothes and diapers; and helping feed, bathe, and attend to personal hygiene, as well as helping nurses chart daily progress, remove catheters, and administer medication. Both hospice positions have given me a deep sense of fulfillment and deepened my longing to be able to serve and treat patients in a greater capacity.

I want to be a PA because I want to be part of a growing profession that is hands-on, practical, challenging, and constantly evolving. Working with supervising physicians means exciting opportunities to acquire new skills and knowledge and the ability to practice in more than one area of health care. With my strong love of learning, a genuine desire to serve patients, and the skills acquired through my life experiences, I feel that I am a strong candidate for the PA profession. If given the opportunity, I also hope to contribute to the PA community by being an advocate for the profession and by helping educate future generations of PAs.

Sample Essay 4

The most powerful experience of my life was when my father was mistreated for Lyme disease, suffered a subdural hematoma, and underwent emergency brain surgery. We were told that his odds were long, but I thank God and the medical team for his full recovery. Above any other, this experience called me to action and motivated me to pursue a career as a physician assistant, where I hope to provide the kind of quality care that my dad received.

My interest in health care and helping others was brewing long before my father's illness, however, and I was raised to work hard in pursuit of my passions. In middle school and high school, I volunteered at a hospital and nursing home, where I relished my interactions with patients as I provided basic care and observed the skilled physician assistants. Though I obviously lacked the technical skills to provide more direct patient care, I learned to build relationships with patients and work alongside medical staff. In college, I directly cared for patients as a personal-care attendant, and I was hooked; I wanted to utilize my skills for the greatest impact.

Given my passion for new experiences, after college I chose a challenging new path. Armed with only confidence, I took a two-year position as a middle-school teacher in a low-income school, where I taught teenagers about their bodies, encouraged budding scientists, and led my students and the science department to success. Surprisingly, it was through this experience that I discovered a new angle on my passion for medicine; witnessing the lack of health care available to these low-income families was my calling to affect change in the medical field. This two-year teaching commitment gave me a deep understanding of the obstacles of the underprivileged and taught me how to educate a reluctant audience while persevering against challenges.

My classroom work was largely external, but in an internal way, my passion for running has impacted my outlook and my attitude on personal health and preventative care. Through college track and running everything from 5ks to marathons, I'm fascinated by the human body. My pursuit of running and wellness has led me to work with friends and family on their personal fitness goals, which has fed my inquisitiveness about the body while improving my ability to educate others on preventative health and wellness. While internal motivation is critical, to gain more direct clinical experience I am now an emergency-room volunteer, where I observe staff making decisions under extreme stress. This exposure has only furthered my desire to pursue a career as a physician assistant.

My journey to pursuing my physician assistant degree has involved events and experiences that have given me tremendous appreciation for the role that PAs play in the health care continuum. I look forward to taking the next step in this journey to serve others.

CONCLUSION

Remember, the essay is probably the most important piece of medical writing that you will ever accomplish. If you need help editing your essay, please visit my website, andrewrodican.com, and sign up for my essay-review coaching package. I've helped thousands of applicants achieve success, and I can help you too.

There are forty sample essays to review in the appendix

Exercise: Create six topic sentences that you may use when writing your essay

Write your sentence after the examples provided for you.

TOPIC SENTENCE 1

Write the first sentence of your essay that will grab the attention of the reader.

(**Example:** *I never had any interest in having a career in health care.*)

_____

_____

_____

_____

Topic sentences 2 and 3: Lead these paragraphs with a topic sentence that will stimulate the interest of the reader (a vignette or example that supports your first paragraph).

TOPIC SENTENCE 2

(**Example:** *In 2014 I traveled to Haiti on a mission to help build houses and provide medical care.*)

_____

_____

_____

_____

TOPIC SENTENCE 3

(**Example:** *I was assigned to work with the medical providers in the makeshift clinic and one critically ill little boy, Les, changed my outlook on the health care profession.*)

_____

_____

_____

_____

_____

TOPIC SENTENCE 4

Use this topic sentence to convince the reader that you are a strong applicant and are motivated to become a PA.

(**Example:** *Having had such a significant emotional experience in Haiti, I feel a career as a physician assistant is the best fit for my goals in life and to serve my community.*)

_____

_____

_____

_____

_____

_____

TOPIC SENTENCE 5

Use this topic sentence to create a desire in the reader to meet you in person.

(**Example:** *My passion for becoming a PA cannot adequately be expressed in five thousand characters or less.*)

_____

_____

_____

_____

_____

TOPIC SENTENCE 6

Use this topic sentence and paragraph to summarize the answer to the question about your motivation to become a PA, and make it one that you feel will seal the deal for you and get you an invitation to interview.

(**Example:** *I may not have started out in my adult life with a desire to become a physician assistant; rather it was my life experiences that led me to this path.*)

_____

_____

_____

_____

_____

CHAPTER 8

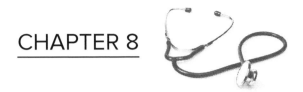

The Interview

THE FIGHT-OR-FLIGHT RESPONSE

I can still remember arriving for my interview at Yale in 1992. My heart was pounding, my breathing was shallow, and I felt like I couldn't remember a thing. Once I met the competition, I felt even more anxiety. Everyone but me had a master's, everyone was more relaxed, and everyone seemed to be more qualified than me.

Once I settled down and practiced a breathing meditation technique I had learned, the anxiety lifted and I was able to perform well enough to be accepted. The key is preparation and relaxation.

Imagine this scenario: You walk out of a building at night, and you suddenly hear the barking of what sounds like a vicious dog. You turn to see a large Doberman pinscher chasing you, with large teeth and foam coming out of his mouth. You immediately go into fight-or-flight mode. You decide to either stay and fight or run. Personally, I would run! Think about what happens to your body's physiology in this type of situation:

- ► Your pulse quickens.
- ► Your breathing becomes shallow.
- ► Your thought process shuts down; now is *not* the time to do equations, balance your checkbook, or answer interview questions!

The following acronym will help you stay calm and relaxed when interviewing. You can even practice this in your car or before you enter the building. It is called the **SHIELD** technique. The SHIELD technique was developed by Eva Selhub, MD (www.drselhub.com). Let's take a look at how to practice this technique whenever you need it:

Stop.
Honor the feeling ("I'm anxious").
Inhale ten times (as if your stomach is a balloon and you are inflating it with your inhalation).

Exhale ten times (as if you are blowing all of the air out of the balloon).

Listen (to what your mind is telling you, for instance, "I'm not qualified enough").

Decide to do something different (focus on the fact that you made it this far, so you do have what it takes to be here).

One way to prepare is to review many of the most common questions that you are likely to be asked at a PA school interview, which are listed later in the chapter. Study them for content and form. Once you do this and become comfortable with the format and what to expect, you can rehearse your own answers and be confident that you will score high at the interview.

Preparation = Improved Confidence = Acceptance

Before we get into the sample interview questions and answers, I would like to touch on a key factor in establishing credibility and inspiring enthusiasm and trust at the interview.

Researchers generally agree that the spoken word is made up of three components: the verbal, the vocal, and the visual. Most applicants focus on the verbal component, but it's the visual component that actually has the most impact. In the visual message, it's the emotion and expression of your body and face as you speak that carry the most weight.

The eye is the only sensory organ that contains brain cells. Research shows that it's the visual image that makes the greatest impact in communication.

The degree of consistency or inconsistency among the verbal, vocal, and visual components of your message determines its believability. The more these three factors harmonize at the interview, the more believable you will be as a candidate. If you send mixed signals, your message may not reach the emotional center of the interviewer's brain, and you won't make that critical emotional connection.

Here are some examples:

▸ You tell your interviewer that you are a trustworthy person, yet you fail to make eye contact during the course of the interview.

▸ You tell the interviewer that you always pay strict attention to detail, yet your suit has a stain on it, or one of your buttons is undone.

▸ You tell the interviewer that you have a lot of passion for becoming a PA, yet you speak in a monotone the entire interview.

▸ You tell the interviewer that you are a very likeable person, yet you never smile during the interview.

> ▶ You tell the interviewer that you have excellent communication skills, yet you persistently use nonwords during the course of your interview: "uh," "um," "like," etc.

Before sitting down for your interview, understanding how the three components of the spoken message are quantified will help you stand out from the crowd. The weights placed on these three components are as follows:

1. Verbal = 7 percent
2. Vocal = 38 percent
3. Visual = 55 percent

As you can see, the visual and the vocal components account for 93 percent of the message. These facts should change the way you think and prepare for the interview. You can answer all of the interview questions perfectly, but if the visual and voice components are off, you won't have a very good chance of scoring high.

I did a mock interview via Skype with a PA school applicant who told me that he interviewed three times in the past year and did not get accepted to any programs. I looked at his CASPA application and was extremely impressed by how good this applicant looked on paper. He had an above-average GPA, thousands of hours of clinical experience as a paramedic, and phenomenal test scores. I was as puzzled as he was.

Less than three minutes into our Skype interview, I told this applicant exactly why he was not getting accepted and why he wouldn't get accepted if he didn't make some changes. He spoke in a monotone, and he rarely smiled. He had a furrowed brow that made him look almost angry. He came off as being too serious, unfriendly, unapproachable, and cold—not exactly the traits of a good PA. I also got the impression that this applicant was probably a loner and would not make a great teammate or classmate. I came to this conclusion in less than three minutes, just by the tone of his voice and the expressions on his face. At this point, it didn't matter how well he answered the questions; he was not a likeable guy. My mind was already made up.

When I called him on these issues, he actually agreed and knew that he didn't present well. Because of his lengthy experience as a paramedic, he dealt with a lot of serious injuries and had to always be focused. It appeared that he was not able to let go of that intense focus. This is why he was getting interviews but not being accepted.

I have interviewed many other applicants who did not know how to use the voice as a powerful tool to make an emotional connection with the interviewer. These applicants spoke in a monotone, which tends to make people sound very boring. Additionally, they appear to have no passion, a key trait to demonstrate when interviewing.

The best way to overcome speaking in a monotone and create passion in your voice is to put your voice on a roller coaster. In other words, try to emphasize at least one word in each sentence, using inflection. For example, "I am extremely *passionate* about the PA profession. My goals are consistent with the *mission* of your program. If I am accepted to this program, I believe I would be a *great* addition to the class."

If you want more examples of how to do this, simply watch news broadcasters when they're on the air. They captivate you and draw you into the story by using inflection and open gestures.

The take-home message here is that you will significantly increase your chances of scoring higher at the interview by simply enhancing the visual and vocal (voice) component of your message: dress appropriately, make good eye contact, smile, avoid facial tics and inappropriate mannerisms, maintain good posture, and put your voice on a roller coaster. Please don't take these suggestions lightly.

I recommend that you obtain a copy of my book, *How to "Ace" the Physician Assistant School Interview*, for correct answers to all of the questions you'll encounter in this chapter.

IDENTIFYING THE KEY ADMISSION REQUIREMENTS FOR PA SCHOOL

The Key Character Traits

The admissions committee is looking for certain traits in strong applicants. I advise that you tailor your interview answers to specifically address these traits as much as possible. Here are six key traits of strong PA school applicants:

1. **Cognitive and verbal ability**
   a. Can you think a problem through and respond appropriately?
   b. Can you articulate your ideas in a logical sequence?
   c. Are you perceptive about others?
   d. Are you organized?
   e. Do you have good time-management skills?
   f. Do you understand and grasp the rigor of the PA program?

2. **Motivation to become a PA**
   a. Are you strongly motivated or just testing the waters?
   b. Are you interested in patients or the "science" of medicine?
   c. Is PA school a stepping-stone to medical school for you?
   d. Have you completed all of the prerequisites?
   e. Do you have medical experience?
   f. Have you shadowed any PAs?

3. **Understanding of the PA profession**
   a. Do you know what PA practice entails?
   b. Have you worked with any PAs?
   c. What is your attitude toward nurses, nurse practitioners, and medical assistants?
   d. Do you understand the dependent nature of the profession?
   e. Do you understand the autonomous nature of the profession?
   f. Do you know the history of the PA profession?

4. **Interpersonal skills and behavior**
   a. Do you work collaboratively?
   b. Do your colleagues and coworkers respect you?
   c. Are you domineering or a team player?
   d. Are you compassionate?
   e. Are you empathetic?
   f. Are you well-groomed?

5. **Ability to handle stress**
   a. Can you be clear, concise, and relaxed at the interview?
   b. What does stress represent to you?
   c. Do you remain poised and relatively calm in the face of stressful situations?
   d. Do you have a sense of humor?
   e. Do you have a measure of self-possession?
   f. Can you think clearly in stressful situations; can you handle the fight-or-flight response?

6. **Personal characteristics**
   a. Are you thoughtful and innovative?
   b. Are the facts you convey in the interview consistent with your experience?
   c. Are you mature?
   d. Are you driven?
   e. Do you have passion?
   f. Are you a motivator?

Knowledge-Based Skills

Some interviewers will look to your knowledge and experience to score you the highest. Others may look at other skills that may be transferrable. Take the time here to identify your own knowledge-based skills. Here are some examples:

- ▶ Compassion
- ▶ Empathy
- ▶ Organization
- ▶ Effective communication
- ▶ Ability to be a team player
- ▶ Leadership
- ▶ Good time management
- ▶ Counseling background
- ▶ Science background
- ▶ Medical background
- ▶ Military background
- ▶ Calmness under fire

Transferable Skills

Transferable skills are important when you might not have medical experience but your experience in other positions has given you many of the skills needed to become a PA. These skills can come in handy when writing your essay or when interviewing.

Keep in mind that most PA programs are not looking to fill a class with a bunch of clones; your unique experiences may be just what is needed to round out an incoming class.

List your transferable skills here. Some examples include communication skills, organizational skills, leadership skills, teaching, coaching, customer service, problem solving, conflict resolution, etc.

Make up your own list:

1. _____

2. _____

3. _____

4. _____

5. _____

Personal Skills

Personal skills are those that make you unique. You cannot teach these skills. You either have them or you don't. My favorite is passion! Other examples of personal skills include high energy, cooperation, calmness, flexibility (going with the flow), empathy, patience, and a sense of humor.

Make up your own list:

1. _____

2. _____

3. _____

4. _____

5. _____

Exercise: The Three Ps

Divide a piece of paper into three columns and label them with the headings "Previous Experience," "Portable Skills," and "Personality Traits." Like the three **P**s of marketing, this will be your PA school marketing tool.

The three **P**'s in Marketing, is a strategy of proven techniques that many companies over the years have developed to become highly profitable in their markets. Following these concepts will guide you to success when selling yourself to the admissions committee

EDUCATION AND PREVIOUS EXPERIENCE

(**Examples:** X-ray technician, medical assistant, retail-store manager, customer-service skills)

1. _____

2. _____

3. _____

4. _____

5. _____

PORTABLE/TRANSFERABLE SKILLS

(**Examples:** Customer relations, communications, time management, organizing skills, analytical nature)

1. _____
2. _____
3. _____
4. _____
5. _____

PERSONALITY TRAITS

(**Examples:** passion, motivation, self-starting nature, friendliness, positive attitude, industriousness)

1. _____
2. _____
3. _____
4. _____
5. _____

When you're done, check each list to see a summary of your accomplishments, traits, and skills that you have to offer. These should match the six key traits that were mentioned on pp. 106–107. The next step is to plan your strategy to show off these traits in the stories you'll need to tell at your interview. Use these traits and stories to convince the committee that you meet the criteria they're looking for.

In the next several pages, we'll be covering the following types of questions you may be asked at your interview:

- ▸ Traditional questions
- ▸ Behavioral questions
- ▸ Ethical questions
- ▸ Situational questions
- ▸ Illegal questions
- ▸ Multiple mini interview questions (MMI)
- ▸ If you were a color/tree/fruit/animal, what would you be? questions

TRADITIONAL INTERVIEW QUESTIONS

Traditional questions are the most commonly asked questions at a PA school interview. They are also the easiest to prepare for since almost every PA program asks similar questions in this format.

The Purpose of Traditional PA School Interview Questions

Traditional interview questions allow the interviewer to get a feel for your

- knowledge of the PA profession;
- reasons for choosing the PA profession;
- personality;
- seriousness as an applicant (are you just testing the water, or are you a serious candidate?);
- communication skills;
- interpersonal skills;
- fitness for the program.

By knowing the most commonly asked questions ahead of time, you will be more confident and less anxious.

Let's start first with the most important question you'll be asked: "Why do you want to become a physician assistant?"

You can count on being asked that question at your interview. I can't tell you how many applicants I've interviewed who look like a deer caught in the headlights when I asked this basic question. I wondered how anyone could go into a PA school interview and be surprised by this question.

I recommend that you prepare your answer to this question and be able to recite that answer as easily as you can recite your date of birth. Be sure not to use clichéd or generalized answers that don't answer the question being asked—statements like "I've always been fascinated by medicine," "I love helping people," or "I'm a people person."

Also remember that the question is asking for an answer as to why you want to become a physician assistant, specifically. It is *not* asking why you want to work in health care. Be sure to answer the question. The clichéd examples above could apply to a desire to become a nurse, a physician, or even a paramedic.

Another thing *not* to do is to recite the American Academy of Physician Assistants' definition of a PA: "PAs are health care professionals licensed to practice medicine . . ." Remember who your audience is—a group of PAs who know the definition of a PA. Additionally, citing the AAPA definition of a PA does not answer the question!

Exercise: Narrow down your answer as to why you specifically want to become a physician assistant

To help you formulate your own answers to these interview questions, I recommend that you answer the following questions:

1. Why don't you want to become a physician?

_____

_____

_____

2. Why don't you want to become a nurse?

_____

_____

_____

3. Why don't you want to become a nurse practitioner?

_____

_____

_____

4. Why don't you want to become a firefighter? They help people too.

_____

_____

_____

By writing down your answers to these questions, you will find it much easier to narrow down your reasons for choosing to become a PA. If your answer to this question describes any of the professions above, you haven't solidified your answer yet.

Sample Questions

In order to help you learn how to answer interview questions effectively, I'll be giving you a round of sample questions in this chapter. I'll also provide three possible answers for each question. Try to select the best answer before looking at the answer key. After you've finished with all of the questions in this chapter, tally the number of correct answers and divide it by the total number of questions to see the percentage of questions you answered correctly.

1. "Tell us about yourself." (Translation: Why are you a good fit?)

Trust me, the interviewer doesn't want to know that you love long walks on the beach. And you're not doing yourself any favors by asking the interviewer what he or she wants to know about you. Consider this an extended version of your elevator pitch, specifically tailored to this opportunity. An **elevator pitch, elevator speech**, or **elevator statement** is a short summary used to quickly and simply define a process, product, service, organization, or event and its value proposition.

The name "elevator pitch" reflects the idea that it should be possible to deliver the summary in the time span of an elevator ride, or approximately thirty seconds to two minutes, and is widely credited to Ilene Rosenzweig and Michael Caruso (while he was editor for *Vanity Fair*) for its origin. The term itself comes from a scenario of an accidental meeting with someone important in the elevator. If the conversation inside the elevator in those few seconds is interesting and value adding, the conversation will either continue after the elevator ride, or end in an exchange of business cards or a scheduled meeting.

Before your interview, review the PA program's requirements and statistics: average GPA, average number of clinical hours for accepted students, first-time pass/fail rate on the boards, clinical rotations, longevity of the program, and the "must haves" to be accepted. Use these top requirements to develop talking points that demonstrate how you are qualified for this program. Weave a story that explains how your experience and skill have led you to this opportunity.

Select the strongest answer to question 1:

(A) *I was born in New England and grew up on a dairy farm. My mother was an X-ray technician, and my father ran the farm. I have three brothers and two sisters. I attended public schools and joined the navy at age seventeen. I was a navy corpsman attached to the Second Marine Division at Camp Lejeune, North Carolina. After an honorable discharge from the navy, I attended Southern Connecticut State University and graduated with a degree in biochemistry. I then went back into the air force as an officer. I currently work as an EMT.*

(B) *I have four years' experience as a navy corpsman and three years' experience as an air-force officer. As a navy corpsman, I often worked autonomously, often under imperfect conditions, and mostly without direct physician supervision. As a junior air force officer, I was often tasked with many projects where I was responsible for up to one hundred subordinates and needed to lead by example. From both experiences I learned to work under stress, I learned to* *exhibit excellent communication and interpersonal skills, and I learned how to be a team player and a team leader.*

(C) *Sure, would you like me to focus on my personal life or my professional life?*

2. "What is your biggest weakness?" (Translation: Prove it. Give me an example.)

Select the strongest answer:

(A) *I believe that we bring about what we think about, so I don't dwell on weakness. However, there was a time recently at work when I came to a realization that I become very impatient with coworkers who don't catch on very quickly to the position. I would sometimes come across as arrogant or frustrated. One day I decided to take one of my coworkers to lunch and find out why I had these feelings. We had a great conversation that sort of melted the ice between us. Right there I realized that I needed to be more of a mentor than a frustrated, angry colleague.*

(B) *I consider myself a workaholic, and I often miss out on family time. I realized that I needed to find more balance in my life, so I now make it a point to go home earlier.*

(C) *My greatest weakness is that I care too much for my patients, and I often go home depressed. I've learned to keep my feelings at work, and I feel much better after work.*

3. Do you have any questions for us? (Translation: How interested are you in attending our program?)

The answer to this question should always be an enthusiastic "Yes," whether you're on your first or third interview that day. Use this opportunity to not only demonstrate your interest and research into the program but to help you better understand the needs of the admissions committee so you can position your skills as the solution to those needs.

Select the strongest answer:

(A) *No, I think we covered everything in the interview.*

(B) *Yes. What are the three most important things you want the applicant who joins this program to achieve during the course of the program?*

(C) *What is this program's first-time pass/fail rate on the PANCE exam?*

ANSWERS TO QUESTION 1

The Strongest Answer

(B) This is the strongest answer because it presents a good summary of what you have to offer. The interviewer knows your total years of experience, the types of places where you have worked, and what you consider your strengths relative to a job. The answer also provides a good blend of knowledge-based skills, transferable skills, and some personality traits. You are striving to give the interviewer a good snapshot of yourself.

The Mediocre Answer

(A) This answer is OK, but it is not as strong as answer **(B)**. This is basically a "summation of your résumé" type answer. "I was born, attended the military, attended college, and worked at…" It would benefit from more detail and specifics, such as types of companies you worked for or some of your strengths and personal characteristics. The ideal answer contains a well-rounded, current picture of you.

The Weakest Answer

(C) This is a very common reply to this question but is a weak answer. It does not show any preparation or planning in regard to what the committee would be interested in knowing about you. Your reply to this question is your opportunity to lead the interview and start out by focusing on what you want the interviewer to know about you and your qualifications for becoming a PA school student. Also, never answer a question with a question.

ANSWERS TO QUESTION 2

The Strongest Answer

(A) This is the strongest answer because it shows that the applicant had the insight that something was wrong with the way he was doing things. He was not getting the results he wanted from his coworkers. By taking one of his colleagues to lunch, he realized the problem wasn't that person, it was him. After becoming aware of his own attitude, he was able to change his outlook, which benefited himself, as well as his colleagues.

The Mediocre Answer

(C) This mediocre answer describes what can be a common problem that many caregivers deal with: they don't know how to leave their feelings at work. It does show some self-awareness, but the answer doesn't really explain how this insight came about.

The Weakest Answer

(B) This answer is fairly clichéd and shows no examples of insight into this problem. It feels canned.

ANSWERS TO QUESTION 3

The Strongest Answer

(B) This answer shows you are interested in the types of applicants who are selected to this program. If you are given an answer to this question in your first interview, you may want to use that answer as fuel when going into your second interview that day.

The Mediocre Answer

(C) This is a good question but one that the applicant should know the answer to before coming to the interview.

The Weakest Answer

(A) This answer shows no interest at all in the program.

Here are four other questions you can ask for question 3:

1. What are the three most important things you want the applicant who joins this program to achieve during the course of the program?
2. If you could describe this program's mission in three words, what would they be and why?
3. What is your vision for this class over the next two years?
4. What kinds of applicants are successful getting accepted into this program?

Here are additional traditional questions to think about:

(Be sure to get a copy of my book *How to "Ace" the Physician Assistant School Interview* for the correct answers to all of the following questions.):

- ▸ Why do you want to become a PA?
- ▸ Why do you want to attend our program?
- ▸ What are your goals as a PA?
- ▸ What do you consider your strengths?

- How would you describe your personality?
- What experience do you have that qualifies you to join our program?
- What do you know about our program?
- What do you value most in a classmate or coworker?
- How have you stayed current or informed about the PA profession?
- If I asked your coworkers or fellow students to say three positive things about you, what would they say?
- If it comes down to you and one other applicant, why should we select you?
- If we remember one thing about you, what should that be?
- Have you applied to other programs? Which ones, and why did you choose them?
- What is a "dependent" practitioner?
- Why do you want to change careers (if applicable)?
- Explain your undergraduate grades.
- If you had a patient with a language barrier, how would you assist the patient?
- What makes you mad?
- Tell us something unique about yourself that's not already included in your application.
- If you could change one thing about the PA profession as you understand it today, what would you change?
- What do you like to do outside of school?
- What fields do you see yourself working in after graduation?
- Tell us your thoughts on health care reform.
- Do you think health-care reform will be a positive or a negative for PAs? Why or why not?
- Should all PA programs be master's-level programs?
- What is the difference between a PA and a nurse practitioner?
- Where do PAs fit on the hierarchy ladder with nurses, nurse practitioners, physicians, and technicians?
- Is it important for PAs to join local, regional, and national associations?
- What do you think the most challenging part of being a PA is going to be?

▸ In your opinion, should PAs be called physician assistants or physician associates? Explain.

▸ What does integrity mean to you?

▸ What is going to keep you from succeeding in this program?

BEHAVIORAL INTERVIEW QUESTIONS

How to Improve Your Interviewing Skills, Particularly with Behavioral Questions

There is an art and a science to conducting a great interview. A great interview goes beyond the standard questions that one would expect and uses various techniques and styles to extract information from the candidate. As a PA you will have to think on your feet and work under stressful conditions. The admissions committee wants to know if you have what it takes to make it through school and be a good ambassador for their program once you graduate.

More and more PA programs are utilizing a technique called *behavioral interviewing*. Interviewers can interpret what you say about yourself and your past behavior as an indicator of how you will behave in the future. In other words, if you did it before, you can do it again. It's in your best interest to be able to demonstrate through the use of recent, relevant examples that you have done similar jobs with proven success. When the interviewer begins to see patterns and hear about successes in your past experiences, you will be considered a serious candidate for admission.

This section focuses on behavioral interview questions. These days, programs are using these types of questions more frequently because they allow the interviewer to find out what specific skills, knowledge, and experience the PA school applicant possesses. Behavioral interview questions can be recognized by the wording used. A typical behavioral question might start with one of the following:

"Tell us about ..."
"Can you give us an example of ... ?"
"Describe a time ..."
"What was the biggest/most important/ most difficult ... ?"
"When was the ... ?"

As soon as you hear the interviewer asking for an example, you should start thinking about telling a *story* as proof that your background on paper supports your claims in real life. The key to understanding behavioral questions is to be specific. The more recent and medically related the example is, the more effective your answer will be.

If you don't have a recent, medically related example to relay, use a volunteer, college, or life experience. The important point is to in some way relate to the qualities sought out in the question.

Using the STAR Technique to Answer Behavioral Interview Questions

The Elements of Your Story

In order to answer behavioral questions, you must tell a story. When asked a behavioral question, you are expected to provide three parts to that story: the **S**ituation or **T**ask, the **A**ction you took, and the **R**esult(s) of that action.

If you memorize this simple acronym, you can use the actual verbiage when giving the answer. This acronym is almost like a cheat sheet for behavioral questions.

Let's examine a behavioral question and an appropriate answer:

"Tell us about a time when you had to handle a stressful situation."

The main clue is to tell the interviewer about a "stressful" situation and how you "had to handle" it. So you must first start by stating the *situation* or *task*. An example response is provided below:

The Situation or Task

The situation was, I was a new air force lieutenant assigned to the 554th Range Group at Nellis Air Force Base, Nevada. One of my first assignments was to travel 250 miles north of Las Vegas to a bombing range in the desert. Fighter pilots from all over the world used this range in an exercise called Red Flag, in which they practiced advanced aerial tactics and bombing wooden targets on the desert floor. We also had live bombing operations going on at different parts of the range.

I was in charge of Coronet Clean, a range cleanup operation that includes carpenters, explosive-ordnance-disposal personnel, and other noncommissioned officers. Our job was to clear the range of unexploded bombs, rebuild the blown-up targets, and do this safely and quickly. This was not easy, as every piece of plywood harbored a sidewinder rattlesnake underneath it—and I'm terrified of snakes!

The Action

The action I took was to meet with my senior noncommissioned officers every morning to make a plan for the day. I touched base with the explosive-ordnance-disposal team to see where they would be clearing bombs. I touched base with the carpenters to see where they would be rebuilding targets. I stayed in touch with the senior noncommissioned officers so they could brief their people. I also had to telecommunicate with headquarters back at Nellis Air Force Base to be sure the range wasn't going to be used for strafing (attacked repeatedly with bombs) by fighter pilots during the times we were working.

The Result

The result was that we accomplished the goal ahead of time, with no casualties, and our unit received a letter of commendation for our efforts. I felt proud that I was a part of that mission.

This answer gets straight to the point and demonstrates a definitive and positive outcome. The goal was accomplished on time, with no casualties, and the interviewee received a letter of commendation.

The interviewer will gain from this story that the applicant can handle stress under fire (literally) and know that the applicant will probably be able to do this again in other situations.

What's Your Story?

Obviously, the above example is very effective. If you are a veteran, you can probably come up with many similar stories. But what if you've never been in the military? What if you're just graduating from college? How do you come up with or compete with a story like that?

The good news is that you don't have to have such a dramatic story. You just need to come up with an answer that will be of interest to the interviewer, and it doesn't have to be medically related.

Exercise: Applying the STAR technique

For this exercise, identify a situation or problem you may have faced where you resolved it, felt good about it, and received praise for it.

_____

_____

_____

Follow the **STAR** technique to answer this same question that you are likely to be asked:

The *situation* or *task*: (what was the problem?)

_____

_____

_____

_____

_____

_____

_____

The *action* you took: (to solve the problem)

_____

_____

_____

_____

_____

_____

_____

_____

The *result* of that action: (in which you were the hero)

_____

_____

_____

_____

_____

_____

_____

_____

Admissions committees are often trying to get a sense of your problem-solving abilities or management style with these types of behavioral questions. When faced with these questions, stick to the STAR approach: describe the situation or task you handled, explain what actions you took to resolve the issue, and summarize the results of your actions, especially how your actions benefited the organization or patient (for instance, streamlined a process, saved the patient's life, helped the team gain better results, etc.). To prepare for the interview, use the core program requirements to brainstorm relevant behavioral questions and succinct stories from your work history that demonstrate your abilities.

1. "Tell us about a time when you had to overcome obstacles to get your job done."

Select the strongest answer:

(A) *In my job, there are always obstacles to overcome. Sometimes a staff member calls out sick, and we have to compensate for that person's duties. Sometimes our physicians are running behind, and we have to effectively communicate with irate patients. A physician's office is a very stressful place to work, and I always have to be flexible to get the job done.*

(B) *I have to work around obstacles all of the time. It's the nature of the job as a medical assistant. One day I have to work around time constraints; the next day it's schedules and deadlines. Of course, I always have people problems to contend with. Every day I plan my day, and then, right when I am getting ahead, some problem occurs. Fortunately, I look at problems as opportunities.*

(C) *I was working as an ER tech in a large inner-city hospital. We received a call from dispatch that a major trauma victim was on his way into our facility. All of our trauma rooms were full. I knew there was an available major-medical room, used to treat patients with serious medical problems—heart attacks, severe dehydration, drug overdoses, etc. I asked the attending physician if we could use the major medical side for this patient, and he agreed. We had to bring in some surgical supplies and struggled a bit to find equipment. However, we were able to improvise and successfully treat the patient.*

2. "Tell us about a time when you had to adapt quickly to a change."

Select the strongest answer:

(A) *I was working as a phlebotomist in a primary-care clinic, when we had a major flu epidemic hit our area. Three of our medical assistants called out sick for the week. Prior to becoming a phlebotomist, I worked as a certified medical assistant. I immediately had to wear two hats—that of a medical assistant and also that of a phlebotomist. I called patients who were scheduled for blood draws and coordinated their appointments for specific, slower times during the week. I worked extremely hard that week, multitasking, but we maintained our patient volume and had not one complaint about waiting times.*

(B) *I actually like change. In fact, I thrive on change. I am a person who can adapt to any situation you put me in. I worked for one internal medicine practice where the office manager changed three times in one year. I didn't let it get to me. I am flexible and roll with the punches. Some people are like oak trees that don't bend very much and will break in a storm. I am more like a palm tree; I go with the flow and bend without breaking. I like being challenged.*

(C) *Change is inevitable. The only certainty in life is change. Change can be frustrating and terrifying at times, but that's how we know we're changing! But change has been really frustrating lately at my current job. There were just too many changes, without any thought behind them. I don't want to complain about management, but sometimes they changed the way we were doing something and the week later changed it back to the way it had been before. That can be very frustrating for an employee.*

ANSWERS TO QUESTION 1

The Strongest Answer

(C) This is the strongest answer because it follows the formula in the STAR technique. It sets up the scene, describes what action the applicant took to treat the trauma patient without compromising care, and indicates that the patient ended up with a favorable outcome. Although the applicant doesn't come out and say, "The situation was . . ., the action I took was . . ., and the result was . . ." she still uses all of the elements of a proper answer to a behavioral question.

The Mediocre Answer

(A) This is not a bad answer if you want to describe some of your positive traits, but it fails to answer the question, "Tell me about a time when . . ." It doesn't pass the STAR technique litmus test.

The Weakest Answer

(B) This is the weakest answer because it has almost a negative tone to it. It does end on a positive note, but it certainly doesn't pass the STAR technique litmus test; it doesn't tell a story.

ANSWERS TO QUESTION 2

The Strongest Answer

(A) This is the strongest answer because it gives a very action-oriented example. There was a problem. The applicant moved quickly to solve the problem. The problem was resolved. There is a strong sense of the applicant's role in the situation. This answer also would be a good reply to a question dealing with problem solving or coming up with a creative idea.

The Mediocre Answer

(B) This answer is not as strong as **(A)**, but it is fairly creative, with a great analogy about the palm tree and the oak tree. However, it would be much better with a specific example of how the applicant specifically dealt with a problem and resolved it.

The Weakest Answer

(C) This answer has a negative, whiny tone. It is not a good idea to bad-mouth former employers in an interview. Even if there were negative circumstances, it is best to let them go in the interview.

Here are twenty-five more behavioral questions to think about:

1. Tell us about a time when you had to handle a stressful situation.
2. Your application states that you're a hard worker. Give us an example of a time when you worked hard.
3. Describe an interaction you've had with a patient who made an impact on you.
4. Tell us about a time when your communication skills made a difference.
5. Give us an example of a time when you took initiative.
6. You mentioned in your essay that you're good at selling new ideas to your boss and coworkers. How do you do that?
7. Tell us about a time when you had a disagreement or confrontation with a boss or coworker.

8. Have you ever been in a situation, at work or in school, where you felt it was necessary to address an ethical issue? Describe the situation.

9. If you and a colleague had a personality clash, what would you do to make it better?

10. Do you think it's important to promote team building in an organization? What steps would you take as a PA student to promote team building in the class?

11. From your perspective, describe what makes a person likeable.

12. Describe a time when you tried your hardest to accomplish something, but you still failed.

13. Talk about a time when you had to work closely with someone whose personality was very different from yours.

14. Describe a time when you struggled to build a relationship with someone important. How did you eventually overcome that?

15. We all make mistakes we wish we could take back. Tell us about a time you wish you'd handled a situation differently with a colleague.

16. Tell us about a time you were under a lot of pressure. What was going on, and how did you get through it?

17. Tell us about the first job you ever had. What did you do to learn the ropes?

18. Describe the most difficult ethical question you've had to deal with.

19. Describe a long-term project that you managed. How did you keep everything moving along in a timely manner?

20. Tell us about a time you set a goal for yourself. How did you go about ensuring that you would meet your objective?

21. Give us an example of a time you managed numerous responsibilities. How did you handle that?

22. Give us an example of a time when you had to explain something fairly complex to a frustrated client/patient/customer. How did you handle this delicate situation?

23. Tell us about your proudest professional accomplishment.

24. Tell us about a time you were dissatisfied in your work. What could have been done to make it better?

25. Tell us about a time when you worked under close supervision or extremely loose supervision. How did you handle that?

ETHICAL INTERVIEW QUESTIONS

Having high ethical standards is a must for anyone who works in the health care profession. As PAs we face ethical challenges every day. We cannot afford to make decisions based on emotion; rather we have to make decisions based on the right thing to do.

You will be asked ethical questions at your interview. You will be given hypothetical scenarios to evaluate, and you will be expected to choose and answer, along with your justification for your choice.

You cannot study for ethical questions and you are not expected to know what it's like to be a PA. However, I will present a few scenarios here to give you an idea what to expect at your interview. There are also many more ethical scenarios presented in my book, *How to Ace the Physician Assistant School Interview*.

Read the questions, and select the strongest answer:

1. "A liver becomes available for a transplant patient, and there are two patients at the top of the waiting list: a sixty-one-year-old female, upstanding member of the community, and a twenty-one-year-old active alcoholic and drug addict. Whom would you choose and why?"

(A) *I would choose the twenty-one-year-old patient because he has a much longer life ahead of him. The elderly member will have this gift for a much shorter period of time.*

(B) *I would interview both of the patients and decide who I think is most appropriate for the liver.*

(C) *I would give the liver to the elderly patient. Although it may seem like the younger patient is the best choice at first, I have to consider his current lifestyle (active alcoholic and drug addict) and his odds of following up appropriately with aftercare and being compliant with his antirejection medications. The fact that he is getting a liver transplant doesn't mean that he is going to stop drinking and using drugs. If he does continue to use alcohol and drugs, the liver won't last very long, and this gift will have been wasted. If he had been clean and sober for a year before I had to make this decision, I might choose differently.*

2. "You are a cardiothoracic-surgery PA. One day you get called down to the emergency department to admit a patient for an immediate cardiac bypass surgery. You meet the patient and begin explaining the risks of surgery, including bleeding. The patient explicitly tells you that she is a devout Jehovah's Witness and her

religion does not allow for receiving blood products of any kind. She is alert and oriented when she tells you this. You document her wishes in her chart. Immediately after the surgery she is brought to the Cardiothoracic Intensive Care Unit, where she begins to bleed uncontrollably. Her blood pressure begins to drop, and she starts going into a fatal arrhythmia. You know that giving blood products would save her life. What would you do?"

(A) *I could not let this woman just die. I would consult with the family first and try to persuade them to allow us permission to give her the blood she needs in order to save her life. I would let them know that she will certainly die without it.*

(B) *I would contact the risk-management department in the hospital. I would explain the situation and see if they would give me permission to give the patient blood products in order to save her life.*

(C) *I would honor this patient's wishes. She made this decision with a sound mind, and it is documented in her chart. Although I would be frustrated that I might have to let this woman die, I would try all other means to save her life.*

3. "You are working in an inner-city clinic. One day a husband and wife are on your schedule to get their HIV test results. The husband is positive for HIV. When he enters your office, you give him the news, and the first words out of his mouth are "Don't tell my wife!" What would you do?"

(A) *I would not tell his wife because of HIPPA laws. I would counsel him on using protection and let him go. That's all I could do.*

(B) *I would not be able to tell his wife because of HIPPA laws. However, I would advise the patient that all STDs, including HIV, are reported to the State Department of Health. I would explain to him that it is their job to call all of the known sexual contacts of the patient, inform them of the results, and advise each of them to get tested for the disease. I would also inform the husband that his wife is going to find out either way. I would ask him if he prefers to have his wife receive a call from a complete stranger, notifying her of his HIV status, or if he prefers to discuss this in the clinical setting, where we can provide HIV counseling.*

(C) *I would feel obligated to tell his wife. After all, HIV could be deadly, and it would be against the law not to tell her. I know about HIPPA laws; however, ethically I could not let this woman leave my office without her knowing her husband's status. At least she would know to use protection when they engage in sexual intercourse.*

ANSWERS TO QUESTION 1

The Strongest Answer

(C) This is the strongest answer because it takes the emotion and the age factor right out of the equation. It is a practical answer that takes into account the lifestyle of the younger candidate and the fact that getting a liver transplant doesn't mean he will stop drinking and using drugs. His liver has been failing for a long time now. If that hasn't motivated him to stop using, why would getting a new liver make a difference?

The Mediocre Answer

(B) Although this answer may seem like the fair thing to do, interviewing both applicants won't change the facts. The alcoholic and drug addict is most likely to destroy this precious gift.

The Weakest Answer

(A) This answer is based on age alone and does not take into consideration the circumstances of both patients.

ANSWERS TO QUESTION 2

The Strongest Answer

(C) You do not have the right to make decisions based on what you think should be done. Although it may be frustrating, you must obey the patient's wishes that she explicitly made known to you before the surgery. Her wishes were even documented in her chart. The decision is out of your hands.

The Mediocre Answer

(B) This seems like a rational approach, and maybe even the correct approach. However, the patient's wishes are clearly documented, so risk management is going to advise you to abide by those wishes and not give any blood products.

The Weakest Answer

(A) This may be how you truly feel, but it is a selfish decision. It would be the same as putting an eighty-year-old woman on life support because you think you could save her life, ignoring the fact that she has a legitimate do-not-resuscitate order in her chart.

ANSWERS TO QUESTION 3

The Strongest Answer

(B) This is the strongest answer because you are not violating HIPPA laws and regulations. You also try to persuade the husband to do the right thing by informing him of the facts. The health department is going to contact his wife anyway. You then offer an alternative way to resolve this problem by offering HIV counseling in the clinical setting.

The Mediocre Answer

(A) At least you don't violate HIPPA laws and regulations in this answer. However, you do very little to offer any alternatives or support. You allow the husband to leave your office without knowledge of his many options. You are almost cosigning his decision.

The Weakest Answer

(C) This answer is a complete violation of HIPPA, period. It may be a noble gesture; however, if we all made decisions based on our emotions, we would take several steps backward in medicine. We would lose the confidence of our patients. Patients would then become cynical and afraid to share information with their health care providers for fear of their spouse or family members finding out.

Here are ten more ethical questions to think about:

1. What do you believe compromises the ethical workplace?
2. Have you worked for a company that had a code of conduct, and did you have positive or negative experiences there?
3. Have you taken a course or had any training in medical ethics?
4. How does being an ethical individual differ from being an ethical corporation?
5. Would you ever lie for us?
6. Tell us about a time that you were challenged ethically.
7. When you've had ethical issues arise at work, whom did you consult?
8. I see you've worked with people from different cultures. What ethics and values did you find you had in common, and where did you differ?
9. Do you believe that all individuals have a right to health care in this country?
10. What would you do if you witnessed a classmate cheating on a test?

SITUATIONAL INTERVIEW QUESTIONS

Responses to situational questions can make or break an interview. An interviewer uses situational interviewing techniques to elicit specific examples of an applicant's ability to perform under stress, work as a team player, and communicate with colleagues. Additionally, the interviewer will want to know how well you understand the role of a PA.

Read the following samples of situational questions and select the best answer:

1. "You are on the hospitalist service in a large medical center. One of the residents writes an order for IV potassium in the chart of a patient you've been taking care of for a week now. You disagree with the order because it may harm the patient. What do you do?"

(A) *I would carry out the order. A resident is higher up than a PA.*

(B) *The first rule of medicine is "First do no harm." I would contact the resident and explain to him why I think this order isn't a good idea. I would engage him in a discussion about his thought process, and I would only carry out the order if I agree with his reasoning over my own. If not, I would not carry out the order, and I would contact the physician hospitalist on the service.*

(C) *I would not carry out the order. If the resident happens to come by again, I would explain to him my reasoning.*

2. "Today you are the first assistant in the operating room for a cardiothoracic surgery case. The patient is already prepped and draped and anesthetized. While you are scrubbing in, the cardiothoracic surgeon enters the room, stumbles, and smells of alcohol. You confront him about the smell, and he tells you that he had a "couple of beers" with some colleagues at lunch. He tells you not to worry about it. What would you do, if anything?"

(A) *I would let the surgeon know that I feel he is impaired. I would tell him that he is jeopardizing the life of the vulnerable patient on the operating table, and I would ask him to voluntarily scrub out of the case. If he refuses, I would inform the anesthesiologist about my concerns and ask her to speak with the physician. If the anesthesiologist allows the physician to continue, I would scrub out of the procedure and inform them both that I am going to call risk management ASAP.*

(B) *Ultimately it is up to the surgeon if he feels he can operate safely or not. I would trust his judgment in this case.*

(C) *I would try to convince the surgeon to scrub out of the case. I would advise him that if he harmed the patient during surgery, and he was found to be intoxicated, he could lose his license. If he reassured me that he was fine to operate, I would assist in the case.*

3. "During one of your clinical rotations, you have a chief resident with a strong foreign accent that you can barely understand. He often uses a patient's illness as a teaching tool, by explaining the concerns you need to have with a patient with that particular illness. He then asks follow-up questions to make sure you understand the key points. Often you don't know what to say because of the communication gap. You also don't feel that you're benefiting from his knowledge because you don't understand what he is saying. What would you do?"

(A) *I would pull the resident aside and tell him that he speaks poor English. I would remind him that I am here to learn and I am paying good money for this experience. I would see if he's willing to change positions with another resident who speaks better English.*

(B) *I would go over the resident's head and ask the supervising physician if he could give us a different resident. I would explain that we cannot understand him and, therefore, we cannot learn what we need to learn on this rotation.*

(C) *I would talk with my group and see if anyone else feels the same as I do. If the group agrees that it is, in fact, extremely difficult to understand the resident, I would ask the group to help me approach the resident and explain the difficulties we are having. I would let him propose a solution. Perhaps he could speak more slowly or ask us if we understand his explanations before we move on.*

ANSWERS TO QUESTION 1

The Strongest Answer

(B) This is the strongest answer because it does follow the first rule of medicine, "First do no harm." However, you also make the appropriate decision to discuss the details of the order with the resident before taking any action. If there remains a disagreement, you decide to contact the physician hospitalist.

The Mediocre Answer

(C) Although you feel strongly about not carrying out the order, you have no communication with the resident who wrote the order. What if the resident knew something that you didn't and you harmed the patient? You may feel this is the right choice in your mind; however, this is not about ego or being right or wrong. It's about the patient, and communication is the key.

The Weakest Answer

(A) This is absolutely the wrong answer. Providers work as a team for the *patients'* well-being. There is no hierarchy when it comes to patient safety.

ANSWERS TO QUESTION 2

The Strongest Answer

(A) This is the strongest answer because you are being an advocate for the patient and trying to stop this surgeon from operating. You follow correct procedure by discussing the situation with the anesthesiologist, who has the ability to wake up the patient and stop the procedure from happening. In the case that the anesthesiologist does not concur with your appeal, you scrub out and contact risk management, who also has the ability to stop the operation.

The Mediocre Answer

(C) This is the mediocre answer because at least you try to get the surgeon to reconsider the operation. You also try to appeal to his sense of responsibility and the fact that he could lose his license. However, you don't take any further action to stop the case, leaving a defenseless patient at risk of injury.

The Weakest Answer

(B) This is the weakest answer. You have no regard for the safety of the patient and don't even try to appeal to the surgeon or anesthesiologist.

ANSWERS TO QUESTION 3

The Strongest Answer

(C) This is the strongest answer because you are going directly to the source and trying to solve a problem. You are also including the rest of the team. The resident is probably aware that he does not speak English well, and he might feel relieved to have a dialogue about this situation. In this case, he may be much more apt to work together with all of you to make changes and improve the quality of your clinical experience.

The Mediocre Answer

(B) Your position may be valid; after all, this is your clinical experience, and you want to make the best of it. However, by going above the resident's head alone, you may cause him to have resentment and compromise the experience for the rest of the team.

The Weakest Answer

(A) Not only is this gesture rude, it will do nothing to solve your problem. You are basically accusing the resident of ruining your clinical rotation. He is not likely to respond well to this kind of confrontation.

Here are fifteen more situational questions to think about:

1. In health care, we deal with all types of patients and coworkers. Explain how you have dealt with a difficult person at work. How did you handle it? What were the results?
2. Describe the work environment where you perform your best work.
3. Please provide an example of an improvement you made at your previous job that made a real difference.
4. What is the biggest challenge you've faced, and how did you solve it?
5. Describe a time when you had to defend an unpopular decision you made.
6. Describe a recent situation where you dealt with an upset coworker or customer.
7. Tell us about your most difficult boss and how you were able to deal with him or her.
8. What would you do if you were working on an important project and all of a sudden the priorities were changed?
9. Please describe a time when your work was criticized by your boss or other coworkers.
10. Share with us a time you went the extra mile to resolve a problem or accomplish something.
11. Team members you've been assigned to lead during a new project object to your vision and ideas for implementation. What specifically would you do to address their objections?
12. You're responsible for an important project near completion but receive another important project that must be completed immediately. How do you multitask and prioritize?

13. When a subordinate is performing below average, what specific steps do you take to correct the problem?
14. You're responsible for ensuring a large amount of work be finished before a school project is due. A classmate decides to use sick time to take an entire week off from school. What would you do to address the problem?
15. What would you do if you knew your supervising physician was absolutely wrong about an important work-related issue?

ILLEGAL INTERVIEW QUESTIONS

Similar to writing good test questions, selecting appropriate interview questions is a skill. Many PA school admissions committee members are not professional interviewers and may not even know what constitutes an illegal question. Questions should be related to your qualifications to become a PA, not to personal information about you, the applicant.

When answering illegal questions, you should ask yourself, "Do I want to be *right* or *effective*?"

Here's the dilemma: if you're asked an illegal question, do you respond, "Hey, that's an illegal question"?

If you absolutely knew that the interviewer knows the question is illegal, you might be tempted to get upset. But what if the interviewer is asking the question out of ignorance? Would you look at the situation from a different perspective?

For the purpose of being effective versus being right, I recommend not answering the question directly. Rather, I pose that you learn to discern the underlying meaning of the question and target your response to it, versus answering the actual question itself.

Review the questions and select the best answer:

1. "Do you have any children?"

(A) *Yes, I have three children.*

(B) *I don't see how the answer to that question relates to my ability to become an effective PA.*

(C) *There is absolutely no reason why I will not be able to show up every day for school and/or clinical rotation.*

2. "You have an interesting accent; what country are you from?"

(A) *That's a very interesting question. Is that information pertinent to my application?*

(B) *I was born in Russia, but I have lived in the United States for the past ten years.*

(C) *I've never been asked that question in an interview. Is that something I have to answer?*

3. "Are you a Republican or a Democrat?"

(A) *I lean to the left on some issues, and I lean to the right on others.*

(B) *I am an Independent.*

(C) *It is my policy never to discuss politics with friends or at an interview.*

ANSWERS TO QUESTION 1

The Strongest Answer

(C) This is the strongest answer because it tells the interviewers exactly what they really want to know: Do you have day care arranged? Will you have to take off any days if your children are sick? So, you've answered the underlying question without answering the actual question being asked.

The Mediocre Answer

(A) This is the mediocre answer because although it is a statement of fact, you may create a doubt in the mind of the interviewer that you may miss days from school or rotations in order to care for your children if needed.

The Weakest Answer

(B) This is the weakest answer because you are really calling out the interviewer. This answer, although it is right, may not be very effective.

ANSWERS TO QUESTION 2

The Strongest Answer

(A) Although you are not specifically challenging the interviewer, you are making him or her think about the purpose of the question. This is not a confrontational answer, and it shows strength on your part.

The Mediocre Answer

(C) This answer starts out OK, but it does challenge the interviewer to make a decision. And what happens if he or she responds yes?

The Weakest Answer

(B) This answer may trigger a bias in the interviewer, and you may be unfairly scored on that question.

ANSWERS TO QUESTION 3

The Strongest Answer

(C) This is a loaded question, and an applicant should *never* discuss the topic. This is the best answer because it puts the interviewer on notice that this topic is off-limits and you are not going to fall into that trap.

The Mediocre Answer

(B) This answer seems like a clever way out of the question. However, you are still setting yourself up for an explanation.

The Weakest Answer

(A) You are hedging your bets on this answer, possibly making it appear that you cannot make a decision.

SCORE YOURSELF

To find out how well you scored, divide the number of your correct answers by thirteen. If you answered over 87 percent of the questions correctly, you have a strong knowledge base on how to answer interview questions. If you scored below 87 percent, you need more practice and a more thorough understanding of how to answer interview questions.

I strongly recommend all applicants invest in my book *How to "Ace" the Physician Assistant School Interview*. This book provides many questions that you may be asked on the day of your interview, including traditional questions, behavioral questions, situational questions, ethical questions, and illegal questions. The book also covers the entire interview process and will certainly give you a competitive edge when it's your turn to complete this final phase of the application process.

I also urge you to invest in my one-hour mock-interview session. You can sign up on my website, andrewrodican.com, under "Coaching Programs." If you feel that you don't have the money to invest in this service, ask yourself, *Can I afford* not *to use this service?* It will take you about two hours to make up this money on your first day of work as a PA.

THE MULTIPLE MINI INTERVIEW (MMI)

What Is a MMI?

A multiple mini interview consists of a series of short, structured interview stations used to assess noncognitive qualities, including cultural sensitivity, maturity, teamwork, empathy, reliability, and communication skills.

Prior to the start of each mini-interview rotation, candidates receive a question/scenario and have a short period of time (typically two minutes) to prepare an answer.

Upon entering the interview room, the candidate has a short exchange with an interviewer/assessor (usually about eight minutes). In some cases, the interviewer observes while the interaction takes place between an actor and the candidate. At the end of each mini interview, the interviewer evaluates the candidate's performance while the applicant moves to the next station. This pattern is repeated through a number of rotations. The duration of the entire interview is usually about two hours.

Generally, the situational questions posed in an MMI touch on the following areas:

- ► Ethical decision-making
- ► Critical thinking
- ► Communication skills
- ► Current health care and societal issues

Although participants must relate to the scenario posed at each station, it is important to note that the MMI is not intended to test specific knowledge in the field. Instead, the interviewers evaluate each candidate's thought process and ability to think on his or her feet. As such, there are no right or wrong answers to the questions posed in an MMI, but each applicant should consider the question from a variety of perspectives.

How Can I Prepare for a MMI?

Candidates typically exhibit anxiety in anticipation of challenging questions that may arise. Many people have difficulty formulating logical, cohesive, polished answers within the allotted preparation time prior to the start of each station.

How well you perform during the actual interview and whether you will ultimately succeed in gaining admission into PA school is in large measure linked to your preparation before the day of the MMI. The most effective preparation is to anticipate the types of questions/scenarios you will face and practice your answers.

Here are a few tips:

1. **Understand the goal:** You should aim to answer the questions in a manner that demonstrates you are capable of being an excellent student and, thereafter, an outstanding physician assistant. Make a list of the attributes that you believe are essential for success, such as integrity and the ability to think critically. Practice integrating these key attributes into your answers.

2. **Work on time management:** Many students experience difficulty with pacing and effectively answering the questions in the allotted time. Remember that once the bell has sounded, the interview must end immediately, even if the candidate is not finished. Therefore, proper pacing is essential. Practice seven-to-eight-minute presentations in advance of your interview to get comfortable with timing. Ensure that you wear a watch that clearly displays the time on interview day, since you cannot rely on a clock being present in each interview room. Appropriately managing your time will give you the opportunity to end the interview in an organized and effective manner.

3. **Listen carefully:** During the MMI, the interviewer will often provide prompts designed to direct you. Listen carefully to the cues provided so you can take advantage of any new information that may be introduced. The prompts may guide you to the specific issues that are the focus of each rotation.

Although success cannot be guaranteed, your performance can improve significantly by learning about the interview process, acquiring strategies to avoid the common pitfalls, and knowing ways to sell yourself so that you get the place you deserve. Poise under pressure can make the difference between achieving your goals and falling just short. As you get ready for the big day, mock interviews should be a key part of your preparations. Simulating what you are about to experience will help build confidence, allowing you to remain calm and more organized on interview day.

Typical MMI Questions

Instructions: Take two minutes to read and consider the prompt. Take eight minutes to answer the prompt (length varies by each university/organization conducting the MMI).

Station #1
PROMPT (read and consider for two minutes):

A close friend in your first-year PA school class tells you that his mother was recently diagnosed with breast cancer. He feels overwhelmed by his studies and is considering dropping out of PA school to spend more time with his mother. How do you counsel your friend?

YOUR RESPONSE (speak for eight minutes).

Station #2
PROMPT (read and consider for two minutes):

Joe is a pizza-delivery worker. The pizza shop he works for guarantees to deliver the pizza within thirty minutes, or else the customer does not have to pay. On Joe's most recent delivery, he spots a woman bleeding on the street. There is no one else around, and the woman seems unable to move by herself. However, Joe knows that if he returns empty-handed again, he will be fired from this job, which he most desperately needs. What do you think Joe should do? Justify your solution in terms of practical and ethical considerations.

YOUR RESPONSE (speak for eight minutes).

Station #3
PROMPT (read and consider for two minutes):

Liberation therapy (LT), a vascular operation developed to potentially cure multiple sclerosis in certain patients, has recently come under very serious criticism, delaying its widespread use. Among other experimental flaws, critics cite a small sample size in the original evidence used to support LT. As a health-care policy maker, your job is to weigh the pros and cons in approving novel drugs and therapies. Please discuss the issues you would consider during an approval process for LT.

YOUR RESPONSE (speak for eight minutes).

Station #4

PROMPT (read and consider for two minutes):

In Canada, because of federal and provincial subsidy policies and return-of-service agreements, international medical graduates (IMGs) now make up an increasingly large proportion of rural doctors. As a consequence, the shortage of doctors in rural areas has prompted many family medicine residencies to increase their quotas for IMGs in their programs. Effectively, this development is leading to a relative reduction in spots available for Canadian medical graduates. Please discuss the pros and cons of such a development.

YOUR RESPONSE (speak for eight minutes).

Station #5

PROMPT (read and consider for two minutes):

Discuss one of your pastimes outside of school and how the skills you acquired from this activity will help you in your career.

YOUR RESPONSE (speak for eight minutes).

Station #6

PROMPT (read and consider for two minutes):

You are a family practice physician assistant seeing Jane, a sixty-seven-year-old woman with a recent history of multiple fragility fractures. You diagnose her with osteoporosis and prescribe some bisphosphonate drugs and other pharmacological treatments. Jane tells you that she has seen some good things on the Internet about alternative-medicine treatments, such as Chinese medicine, and she is adamant on trying these as well. You are concerned about the use of these alternative-medicine treatments and the possible negative effects they could have on Jane's health. How would you handle the situation, and what would you recommend Jane do? Discuss any ethical considerations that are present.

YOUR RESPONSE (speak for eight minutes).

Station #7

PROMPT (read and consider for two minutes):

You are on the committee for selecting a new dean of science. What characteristics and/or qualities would you look for when selecting an effective dean?

YOUR RESPONSE (speak for eight minutes).

Station #8

PROMPT (read and consider for two minutes):

In June 2011, the infamous Vancouver riots took place after the city's hockey team lost in the Stanley Cup Finals. Stores were ransacked, and cars were burned. Hundreds of people were injured and sent to overcrowded hospitals. As the police chief in Vancouver, what measures or policies would you put in place to make sure this did not happen again?

YOUR RESPONSE (speak for eight minutes).

Station #9

PROMPT (read and consider for two minutes):

Clostridium difficile is a type of bacteria that increases its activity with most antibiotic use and is, therefore, very difficult to treat. Research shows that the most effective way to prevent the spread of infection is frequent hand washing. However, many people have flat-out refused to wash their hands in hospitals. The government is contemplating passing a policy to make it mandatory for people entering hospitals to wash their hands or else risk not being seen by doctors and being escorted out of the building against their will. Do you think the government should go ahead with this plan? Consider and discuss the legal, ethical, or practical problems that exist for each action option, and conclude with a persuasive argument supporting your decision.

YOUR RESPONSE (speak for eight minutes).

Station #10

PROMPT (read and consider for two minutes):

Discuss an experience that allowed you to learn something important about yourself. How will this lesson help you succeed in your career?

YOUR RESPONSE (speak for eight minutes).

PA-SCHOOL INTERVIEW QUESTIONS AND ANSWERS

"If You Were an Animal/Color/Fruit/Tree, What Would You Be?"

It is becoming increasingly common for interviewers to throw in some unusual questions during interviews rather than sticking to the tried and true. This could be for a number of reasons: they want to see if you can think on your feet, think creatively, say something illuminating about yourself, and, possibly, demonstrate a sense of humor.

This trend can take the form of a question such as "If you were an animal, what would you be?" Variations of this kind of question could include, "If you were a fruit, what would you be?" or even "If you were a breakfast cereal, what would you be?"

There is obviously no right answer to questions like these, nor can you plan for them, but this is your chance to be creative and really impress with your inventiveness. What is required is for you to think fast, not get flustered, and try to think of something that represents your best attributes that are also attributes of a strong PA school applicant.

For example, when it comes to animals, do you exhibit the loyalty and friendliness of man's best friend, the solid work ethic of an ox, the industriousness of a beaver, or the cleverness and sociability of a chimp? If you're a person who pays strict attention to detail, perhaps you have the acute eyesight of an eagle, able to swoop in on the smallest spelling or typographical errors while also keeping your eye on the big picture from above. Whatever your choice, try to choose an animal with generally positive associations.

When it comes to fruit, almost anything will do as long as you can give a good reason for it. You can choose a fruit that goes well in a fruit salad to show that you're a team player and get along with others…or a banana, which is versatile, transportable, and has substance…or something a bit different, like a tomato, which crosses the line between fruit and vegetable, is highly versatile, and can be eaten raw or cooked, all traits demonstrating flexibility and transferability of skills.

"If You Could Be Any Color, What Color Would You Be?"

You should approach this question, as well as any question asking you to pick something to represent you, as a way for the admissions committee to gain insight into your personality. Never answer the question with a random color you have picked simply because you like it or it's pretty. This tells the interviewer nothing about you, apart from the fact that you seem uninteresting and uncreative.

Tailor your answer to the PA profession, and the more creative you are the better. A good color to choose to demonstrate that you can work in a stressful environment could be blue: it implies that you keep your cool and never lose your head in high-pressure situations.

Choose colors that highlight your best qualities, and make sure you justify why you chose that color. Using colors that have warm and friendly connotations are great, but don't be afraid to pick colors that are unusual—remember there are many shades to the color wheel.

For example, you could say that you would be a darker shade of charcoal gray because you're an efficient and quiet worker, a warm person (because darker colors absorb heat from the sun while lighter colors deflect heat), and you think gray is a chic, understated color that can complement other colors.

Like other quirky questions, there is no "right" answer, so feel free to take things whichever way you want. What you will be judged on is creativity and your analytical and problem-solving abilities.

"If You Were a Tree, What Would You Be?"

Perhaps you would be an oak tree, standing tall and strong, or perhaps you would be a palm tree that is very flexible and won't break in the midst of a severe storm: it's resilient and rides out the storm intact.

Remember, there is no right answer to this sort of question; it's all about trying to see your thought processes, how you handle being put on the spot, and your ability to be a little creative. Try to tailor your answer to the specific requirements needed to become a PA.

CHAPTER 9

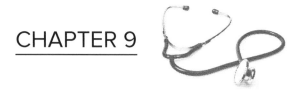

Putting It All Together

At this point you may be feeling a bit overwhelmed. I don't blame you. It takes a lot of hard work, determination, and research to become a competitive applicant for PA school. If you did the work in this book, however, you are now a much stronger applicant for having done so. In this chapter I will attempt to cover the salient points of the book and motivate you to *do the work* (if you haven't) and reach your goal of getting into the PA school of your choice.

HISTORY OF THE PA PROFESSION

Learning as much as you can about the PA profession and its roots will provide you with a much higher comfort level when completing the entire application and interview process. The admissions committee will know if you've done your homework or not. As a former admissions-committee member, I can tell you it becomes blatantly obvious during the course of your interview(s) if you have a firm grasp on the history of the profession. The more you know about the profession, the higher you will move up on the list of strongest applicants.

To keep this really simple for you, I will provide you with several websites and suggestions. These websites will provide you with plenty of history about the PA profession, including current events relative to the profession.

The following is a list of recommended websites to explore:

The American Academy of Physician Assistants' website, www.aapa.org

The AAPA website provides the following information:

Every applicant should become intimately familiar with this website and join this organization as an affiliate member. The American Academy of Physician Assistants (AAPA) is the national professional society for PAs in the United States. It (currently) represents approximately 104,000 certified PAs across all medical and surgical specialties in all fifty states, the District of Columbia, all US territories, and within the uniformed services.

AAPA advocates and educates on behalf of the profession and the patients PAs serve. It works to ensure the professional growth, personal excellence, and recognition of physician assistants and to enhance PAs' ability to improve the quality, accessibility, and cost effectiveness of patient-centered health care.

The AAPA was established in 1968, and its first group of members included students and graduates from the first PA program, Duke University.

In 1973, the organization had three hundred members and established joint national headquarters in Washington, DC, with the Association of PA Programs, which is now the PA Education Association (PAEA). The headquarters moved to Arlington, Virginia, in the late 1970s and then to Alexandria, Virginia, in 1988.

PAs who are graduates of PA educational programs accredited by the Accreditation Review Commission on Education for the PA (ARC-PA) or one of its predecessor agencies are eligible for fellow membership in the AAPA. Other membership categories include the following:

- ▸ PA students and pre-PA students
- ▸ Physicians
- ▸ PAs who are no longer practicing but wish to support the profession
- ▸ Related health professionals and service providers

Volunteer leaders (elected and appointed) and paid staff serve the profession from the national office headquarters in Alexandria and other US locations. There are other divisions of the AAPA:

- ▸ **The Student Academy** is dedicated entirely to students completing an accredited PA program.
- ▸ The **PA Foundation** is the organization's philanthropic arm, fostering knowledge and philanthropy that enhance the delivery of quality health care.
- ▸ The **Association of Family Practice PAs** is an organization that represents and advocates for PAs in primary care and family practice where the greatest need is in health care.

The AAPA provides the following services:

- ▸ **Advocacy and government affairs**—AAPA's advocacy staff lobbies policy makers and third-party payers at both the federal and state levels to support PAs' ability to deliver quality health care with minimal barriers and practice to the level of their licensure.

▶ **Reimbursement and information**—AAPA reimbursement staff work to ensure that insurance companies and other third-party payers cover PA-provided medical and surgical services.

▶ **Education and professional development**—AAPA is a resource for continuing medical education (CME) and provides PAs with a vast number of continuing-medical-education resources, such as its yearly Cleveland Clinic conference for PAs in clinical management and conference. The professional-affairs staff works with PAs on issues such as credentialing, privileging, the Joint Commission, liability insurance, contracts, compensation, and benefits to secure professional standing and free PAs to focus on patient care.

▶ **Public-awareness building**—AAPA actively promotes the value of PAs to patients, physicians, and the general public through comprehensive marketing and communications campaigns.

▶ **Research**—In partnership with PA-focused organizations, AAPA collects data on the profession and analyzes and publishes its findings. AAPA also produces original research that demonstrates the critical role PAs play in high-quality, accessible patient care. It produces an annual census and salary report.

▶ AAPA delivers information for and about PAs through both print and online publications, including *PA Professional* and *JAAPA* (AAPA's scholarly, peer-reviewed journal).

▶ **Partnership with constituent organizations**—Constituent organizations are independent organizations that AAPA officially charters or recognizes. These organizations are grouped into four categories and include chapters, specialty organizations, caucuses, and special-interest groups.

▶ **Community outreach/public health**—AAPA also works with foundations run by PAs and partners on public-health initiatives and awareness campaigns, such as the Horse Rhythm Foundation, the Long Road Home Project, and the National Interprofessional Initiative on Oral Health.

AAPA State (Constituent) Chapters' website, aapa.org /about_aapa/constituent_organizations/chapters/

AAPA's constituent chapters—based within five regions (for state chapters) and five federal service areas—provide their members locally based CME, networking opportunities, social gatherings, timely information, advocacy, and job resources. **Be sure to join your state chapter of the AAPA.**

AJR Associates' website, andrewrodican.com

This is my own personal website where I provide several free resources, including a complete list of all of the PA programs' websites. Additionally you can purchase all of my books on this site and sign up for my one-on-one services, like essay review and edit, mock interviews (via Skype), and one-on-one coaching (via Skype).

AJR Associates' Facebook page, facebook.com/ajrassociates

I personally update this page with information that is exclusively relevant to PA-school applicants. This is a great resource to keep up with current events relative to the PA profession. I also provide frequent tips on everything from the application process through the interview.

The Physician Assistant Education Association's (PAEA's) website, paeaonline.com

The PAEA is the only national organization representing physician assistant educational programs in the United States. Currently, all of the accredited programs in the country are members of the association. PAEA provides services for faculty at its member programs, as well as to applicants, students, and other stakeholders.

The association was founded in 1972 as the Association of Physician Assistant Programs. Member programs voted to adopt the current name in 2005. You can find a searchable directory of member PA programs on my website, andrewrodican.com, or you can go to the PA Programs Directory (directory .paeaonline.org)

The Centralized Application Service for Physician Assistants' (CASPA's) website, www2.paeaonline.org

This website can be found on the PAEA website. The Central Application Service for Physician Assistants is a full-service, web-based application system that will allow students to apply to multiple participating PA educational programs with a single application, as well as facilitate a streamlined admissions process for programs.

PAs Connect blog, pasconnect.org

PAs Connect is an online community for PAs to communicate, learn, share their experiences, and discuss changes in the profession. It also seeks to educate the public about the PA profession and promote awareness. The site features stories, a student section, a forum, and a blog.

Physician Assistant History Society's website, pahx.org

The Society for the Preservation of Physician Assistant History, Inc. (PA History Society) is dedicated to the history and legacy of the physician assistant profession through the identification and collection of appropriate papers, manuscripts, magazine and newspaper clippings, newsletters, reports, dissertations, oral histories, and visual artifacts, such as films, videos, photographs, and digital images.

The PA Forum, physicianassistantforum.com

The PA Forum is an excellent resource for physician assistant school applicants. Although there are many individual forums on the site, there is a specific forum dedicated to PA school applicants, "Pre-PA," where you can post questions and read posts from other applicants. The "Pre-PA" section includes the following forums:

- ▸ Pre-PA general discussion
- ▸ Physician assistant schools
- ▸ CASPA
- ▸ Personal statements

The *Journal of the American Academy of Physician Assistants'* (*JAAPA's*) website, JAAPA.com

JAAPA is the official journal of the AAPA. It is published on a monthly basis and contains clinical articles, as well as articles relevant to current events, job opportunities, and other information on current hot topics in the PA profession. When you join the AAPA, you will automatically receive this journal.

If you follow my recommendation to visit these websites and join the AAPA and your state chapter of the AAPA, you will have access to a plethora of information on the PA profession at the state and national level and your knowledge of the PA profession will be unparalleled to the majority of PA school applicants.

Do the work!

WHY DO YOU WANT TO BECOME A PHYSICIAN ASSISTANT?

This is the million-dollar question that so many PA school applicants struggle with when writing the essay and answering this question at the interview. Here are some common mistakes applicants make when answering this question:

1. **Not answering the question being asked.** Remember, the question is not asking why you want to work in health care; the question specifically asks why you are choosing the PA profession over all other medical professions.

2. **Repeating everything already listed in your CASPA application (your résumé).** Why would you want to repeat information that the admissions committee already knows about you? You only have five thousand characters to provide a concise answer to this question, so don't waste precious real estate by telling the committee what they already know.

3. **Not taking the time to think about how you became motivated to choose this career path.** You may have to invest the time to do some soul-searching to determine exactly what motivated you to decide to pursue a career as a PA. The time you invest to do this will pay off appreciably.

It is very obvious to the admissions committee when an applicant hasn't taken the time to reflect on the *real* answer to this question. The committee will read thousands of essays per year and interview over a hundred applicants. It quickly becomes evident who is a serious applicant—one who has put a lot of effort and thought into choosing this profession, versus the applicant who is just *testing the waters* to see if he or she can get into PA school doing the minimal amount of work.

Applicants who choose to follow the common path and not do the work necessary to answer this question are the ones who use cliché answers like

- ▶ *I've always been fascinated by medicine;*
- ▶ *I've known I wanted to work in health care since I was five years old;*
- ▶ *I love helping people;*
- ▶ *I'm a people person;*
- ▶ I'm a team player.

If you think about it, all of these statements could be answers to why you want to become a nurse, a fireman, a physician, a nurse practitioner, or an EMT.

Write down your answer to why you want to become a PA, and after reading through it, if your answer could be applied to any one of the professions above, you have not completely answered the question. Using this technique will be your litmus test to see if you've properly answered the question "Why do you want to become a physician assistant?"

SELECTING A PA PROGRAM

Selecting a PA program that will be a good fit for your qualifications will take a little research and a lot of honesty. You will have to visit the websites of the programs you are interested in and review the admissions criteria to see where you stand. If you fall short of some of these qualifications, you may be tempted to bury your head in the sand and apply anyway. If you do this, you will be making a fatal mistake.

My recommendation to those applicants who fall short of the admissions criteria, even if it's just by one class, is to wait another year to complete that class, increase their medical experience, and do whatever it takes to exceed those admissions criteria.

I strongly recommend that you refer back to chapter 3 to review the average GPA, test scores, and health-care experience of first-year applicants. This will be a good reality check, and hopefully you'll realize the importance of strengthening your application.

Exercise: How do you pick the PA programs you want to attend?

If you make it to the interview, one of the questions that you are likely to be asked is, why have you selected our program? From my personal experience on the admissions committee at Yale and from my many years of doing mock interviews with PA school applicants to every program in the country, I find that many answer this question in the following manner:

> I like the fact that Emory is looking for diversity in its applicants. I also like the fact that Emory emphasizes evidence-based medicine with a focus on primary care. I like the focus on teamwork and that the Emory PA program supports team-based practice. Finally, Emory has a great reputation as one of the best PA programs in the country, and since Emory is only a thirty-minute drive from my home, I will be able to commute to school every day.

Compare that answer to this one:

> *I am applying to Emory because the program has a 93–98 percent first-time pass/fail rate on the Physician Assistant National Certification Examination. Emory is also consistently ranked as one of the top five PA programs in the country (currently ranks number three). I know that if I graduate from Emory, I will be able to pass my boards and immediately begin working as a physician assistant. I appreciate the rich history and longevity of Emory's PA program, which has been educating PAs since 1971. I'm comfortable that all of the "kinks" have been worked out over the years, both academically and clinically, to provide the highest-quality educational experience. Emory's PA program is also affiliated with the Emory medical school, which is a great resource for PA school applicants. I also like the fact that Emory has a cadaver lab, so students don't have to learn anatomy on plastic models.*

Notice that the first answer is not very specific to Emory's PA program, except for the reputation of the program. The first few sentences hold true for the majority of PA programs in the country. Geography is OK to mention, but there are many more important reasons to choose a PA program besides convenience.

The second answer gets very specific:

- *First-time pass/fail rate of 93–98 percent on the Physician Assistant National Certification Examination*
- *Consistently ranked as one of the top five PA programs in the country*
- *Affiliated with the Emory medical school*
- *Has a cadaver lab*
- *Longevity, began training PAs in 1971*

The take-home message here is to gather the facts and provide specifics when answering the question, "Why have you selected our program?"

Exercise: Complete the following chart for all of the PA programs you are considering

PA Program	
Year Started	
1st Time Pass/Fail Rate on PANCE	
Current Ranking (nationally)	
Affiliated with a medical school?	
Cadaver lab?	

After filling in this table for all of the programs you plan to apply to, and after completing exercise on pp. 151–152, you will now be armed with the information you need to make an informed decision about the PA programs that will be the best fit for your qualifications. And you will have no trouble when you are asked, *why have you selected our program?*

COMPLETING YOUR PERSONAL GOAL SHEET

Yogi Berra once said, "If you don't know where you're going, you might not get there." How true. If you were a sailor and your goal was to sail from New York City to Naples, Italy, you would certainly plot a course before you left and bring along a compass to keep you on course. Along the way you would have to make corrections in your course to get you exactly to the right port.

The same principle is true for applying to PA school. You must have a specific plan to get you into the program of your choice. All of the things that need to be a part of that plan are covered in this workbook. And if you complete the exercise above, you will have a specific order in which to accomplish each mini goal. You simply need to set deadlines for each of these mini goals until you've accomplished them all.

Along the way to accomplishing your goal of getting into PA school, you will also have to adjust your path. You may decide to repeat another science class in which your grade was poor. You may decide to retake your GREs or obtain more health-care experience. Whatever it is that you need to do, by having a goal and a plan, all you have to do is follow your road map to success.

In the chapter called "Completing Your Personal Goal Sheet," I give you a specific example of how to develop your personal plan of action to get into the

PA school of your choice. If you've completed that exercise, you are already far ahead of the competition.

In this section, I would like to reinforce the importance of having a specific goal committed to in writing and advise you how to use the technique of imaging to dramatically increase your odds of achieving any worthy goal in life.

William Arthur Ward once said, "If you can imagine it, you can achieve it. If you can dream it, you can become it." In this quote he is speaking specifically to the technique of imaging.

One example of using imaging to accomplish a goal is to create a vision board. I personally have a vision board to help me achieve everything on my "bucket list" of things I'd like to accomplish and places I'd like to visit in my life. This board is in my office, and it is filled with pictures and articles on my short-term and long-term goals in life.

For example, one of my goals in life, after retirement, is to purchase a recreational vehicle (RV) and travel to every state in the country (except Alaska and Hawaii of course), focusing on all of the major parks and monuments. I have a picture of the exact RV I want to purchase and a map of the United States with pins in the exact locations of the sites I want to visit in each state. I have pictures, articles, and diagrams for every item on my bucket list, which helps me visualize each experience. Looking at this board daily keeps me focused on the goal and sends the message to my subconscious mind to get working on plans to make it happen.

THE APPLICATION PROCESS

PA school applicants should take the application process very seriously and pay strict attention to detail when achieving each task along the way. Think of preparing a PA school application as a second job. Make it a point to know everything there is about the PA profession, the programs you are choosing, and the CASPA application itself. Be sure to give yourself enough time to do your homework. Everyone wants to apply to PA school yesterday, but you must first learn many things before you apply.

Here are ten steps you need to take if you want to be a serious, competitive applicant:

1. Learn about the history of the PA profession using the resources I've listed for you in the website section of this chapter.
2. Join the American Academy of Physician Assistants as an affiliate member and also join your state chapter of the AAPA.

3. Keep up with current events and topics relative to the PA profession by reading the *Journal of the American Academy of Physician Assistants* (*JAAPA*) and by attending state chapter monthly meetings.

4. Visit each program's website where you plan to apply, and read every section on that website, including the biographies of the staff and faculty.

5. Continue to gain health care experience and retake any science classes that you feel necessary to strengthen your application.

6. Create a CASPA account, and begin reading through the CASPA application process. Be sure to write down deadlines for all of the items you need to accomplish and check them off as you go. Please pay strict attention to detail, and follow the instructions as written.

7. Find three solid people who know you well and will agree to write a strong and positive letter of recommendation for you. Write the letters yourself, and use the phrases provided in the chapter titled "The Letter of Recommendation."

8. Write several drafts of your essay. Be sure that your essay answers the question being asked concerning your motivation to become a physician assistant versus a health-care provider. Have your essay reviewed by several people or sources, such as my essay review and editing service located on my website.

9. Purchase my book *How to Ace the Physician Assistant School Interview* and begin reviewing the different types of interview questions and scenarios. Consider doing a one-on-one (Skype) mock interview with me. You can also sign up for this service on my website.

10. Remember this quote by Ben Franklin: "By failing to prepare, you are preparing to fail."

THE LETTER OF RECOMMENDATION

Obtaining strong letters of recommendation (LORs) may or may not increase your chances of being invited to interview. However, if any of your LORs are negative ("Jim rarely pays attention to detail"), it can ruin your chances of getting invited to interview. So the take-home message is to follow some simple steps to ensure that your LORs will contain strong and positive content about your candidacy for applying to PA school.

Refer back to chapter 4 and review the tips I provide on obtaining a perfect LOR.

THE ESSAY

The essay is your ticket to the interview. Even if your GPA or health-care experiences fall a bit short of the most competitive applicants, writing a persuasive essay that creates an emotional connection with the reader may create just enough interest to persuade the reader that he or she would like to meet you in person to find out more about you.

On the other hand, if you have the most competitive GPA, health-care experience, and test scores, yet fail to make that emotional connection with your essay, you may not be invited to interview.

I've covered a lot of information about writing the CASPA essay in all of my books, and I provide forty sample essays in the appendix at the end of this book.

Let's now focus on the basics of writing a good essay, in general.

1. **Read the question:** *Please explain why you are interested in being a physician assistant.*

   The question is not asking why you want to work in health care. The question is asking, specifically, why you want to be a PA. If you write your essay and you can substitute the words physician assistant with nurse, physician, EMT, or nurse practitioner, chances are you haven't answered the question.

   Be sure to do your homework. Read the essays in the bonus chapter at the end of this book. DO NOT plagiarize any of these essays, but get a feel for what a well written essay might look like. All of the applicants who wrote these essays received an invitation to interview.

2. **Grab the attention of the reader in the first sentence or paragraph.**

   Your opening sentence must be unique and interesting in order to draw the reader into your essay. Support the opening sentence with a vignette if you can. By telling a story, you can personalize the essay and demonstrate to the reader that you are a real person.

   Avoid using cliché openings like, *I knew I wanted to work in health care since I was five- years old, or, I love helping people.* Admissions committee members will read hundreds of essays during the course of an application cycle. If your essay starts out with a cliché, it's likely to be placed to the side and probably not even read.

3. **Create interest.**

   This is your essay and it should be personal to your experiences.

   The best way to create interest in an essay is to tell a story, or vignette, to keep the reader interested. Using vignettes personalizes your essay and convinces the reader that you have your own unique reasons for choosing to become a PA.

Make sure that your essay doesn't read like your resume. If you traveled on a mission to help build houses in Haiti, explain how that experience impacted you. Was there a certain person, child, or family that opened your eyes to a new way of looking at the world? Did you learn something insightful about yourself in the process?

Take the time to brainstorm ideas and insights you've gained from your personal experiences. Show that you are a real person, with your own unique experiences that make you the person you are today and how these experiences have shaped your desire to become a PA.

4. **Show conviction.**

Use the essay as a tool to show the admissions committee how you became specifically convinced to become a physician assistant versus any other health-related career. Spend a lot of time thinking about the exact moment you knew that becoming a PA was what you wanted to do. If you don't present compelling evidence that you've thought about the PA career field and you have a definitive reason for choosing it, you will not score many points with the reader.

5. **Create desire.**

Never forget that the essay is your ticket to the interview.

The sole purpose of your essay is to persuade the reader to have a desire to meet you in person. You can even overcome poor grades or lack of experience by writing a compelling essay. Leave the reader with no doubt that becoming a physician assistant is your number one goal in life and that you are pursuing this goal with a passion.

6. **Close the deal.**

Your closing paragraph should be a strong reiteration of why you want to become a physician assistant. Leave no doubt that this career field is a perfect match for your goals in life and that you have the qualities, experience, and compassion to make a great PA. Let the reader know that you're not just "testing the waters.", rather you're a serious applicant who deserves to have an interview to make your case.

THE INTERVIEW

I received an e-mail a few months prior to this writing from a gentleman I'll call John. I could tell from his e-mail that he felt desperate and frustrated. John advised me that he just received an invitation to interview at a PA program and he was very concerned. He went on to explain that this was his third year in a row interviewing at various PA programs and he could not figure out why he wasn't being accepted. I asked him to e-mail his CASPA application to me, and he signed up for a mock interview via Skype. I told him that we would figure it out together during our interview session.

When I reviewed John's CASPA application, I was totally baffled. He had a 3.8 GPA, he was a former navy SEAL with five thousand hours of health-care experience as a medic, and he wrote an extremely compelling essay. I thought to myself that this guy has one of the most competitive applications on paper that I've ever reviewed. I e-mailed him back before the mock interview telling him so and reassured him that he must be doing something wrong at the interview.

The night of the scheduled mock interview, I prepared my computer and called him on Skype. When we connected, I saw this very fit, well-groomed man who had the initial appearance of a serious applicant.

After exchanging pleasantries, I began asking John some routine questions about his CASPA application, where was he interviewing, where had he interviewed in the past, and why he thought he had not been accepted to any of these programs. During the course of this brief conversation, I began to notice that something was off. I couldn't immediately place my finger on what exactly was wrong, but I knew I would figure it out during the course of the interview.

It only took about five minutes into the interview before I figured out the problem. John was still in military mode. He never smiled, he spoke in a monotone, and he was very stiff and almost appeared to be a little frightening. His answers to the questions were spot-on, but his monotone voice, intimidating appearance, and lack of emotion were his problem. I advised him of this, and he nodded in agreement as if he knew this was his problem.

Throughout the course of the mock interview, I taught John a crucial
**mittee selects applicants based on an emotional
r decision with the facts.** Even though the fact was
candidate on paper and even though he knew the
e questions, he failed to make an emotional connec-
ring the course of the Skype session, I educated John
led to acquire to become a more likeable candidate. I
to loosen up a bit. We discussed eye contact and using

inflection in his voice so his message would be much more interesting. I never heard back from John, and I hope he performed well.

So, how do we make that emotional connection at the interview? We need to understand that the spoken message is made up of three components:

1. The verbal component
2. The vocal component
3. The visual component

Professor Albert Mehrabian has pioneered the understanding of communications since the 1960s. He quantifies the spoken message in the following way:

- ▸ Seven percent of a message pertaining to feelings and attitudes is in the words that are spoken.

- ▸ Thirty-eight percent of a message pertaining to feelings and attitudes is in the way that the words are said.

- ▸ Fifty-five percent of a message pertaining to feelings and attitudes is in facial expression.

Given this information, we can now understand why John is not getting accepted to PA school. Although he scores high in the spoken message, or the words he uses to answer the questions at his interviews, he scores extremely low in the two most important areas of spoken communication; the vocal message (using inflection and intonation) and the visual message (facial expressions and open gestures.).

John fails at 93 percent of his spoken message.

If you want to score high at your interview, you must be consistent with all three elements of your spoken communication that day. The more these three factors harmonize, the more believable, likeable, and trustworthy you will be as an applicant. If your verbal message is not in harmony with your body language, you send a mixed signal to the emotional center of the interviewer's brain. Your message may or may not get through to the decision-making, rational portion of the brain.

Here are eight (strong) recommendations to enhance your message at the interview:

1. **Make eye contact**. This is the number one skill you should develop before your interview. There are three rules for maintaining eye contact:

   - ▸ Use involvement rather than intimacy or intimidation. In other words, don't stare anyone down, and be sure to make eye contact with all of the interviewers if you're in a group format.

- ► Count to five (involvement) and then look away.
- ► Don't dart your eyes; this represents a lack of confidence.

2. **Utilize good posture and movement.** Good posture commands attention, and movement shows confidence. Walk into the room standing tall. Don't slump. When you speak to your interviewer, don't be afraid to add movement to your message. Do this by using open gestures to come across as friendly and open-minded.

   Here are four rules for posture and movement:

- ► Stand tall.
- ► Watch your lower body; don't lean back on one hip or rock back and forth.
- ► Get in the ready position; lean slightly forward if you're sitting or on the balls of your feet if you're standing.
- ► Use movement to show that you're excited, passionate, and confident.

3. **Wear a suit.** The third way to enhance your message is with dress and appearance. **You get only two seconds to make that critical initial impression.** If you blow it, it may take more than thirty minutes to recover, and most interviews last only twenty minutes. So, it is critical to make a good first impression.

   When you dress up for an interview, only 10 percent of your skin should show. Be sure that your face is well shaven or your makeup is not too overbearing. Comb or style your hair, avoid wearing extravagant jewelry, clean and trim your nails, and use cologne or perfume sparingly.

   Here are five rules to remember when it comes to dressing for the interview:

- ► Be appropriate—when in Rome . . .
- ► Be conservative; when in doubt, dress up.
- ► Men, always button your jacket.
- ► Don't overkill cologne or perfume.
- ► Always check yourself in a mirror before you walk into your interview.

4. **Use open gestures and smile.** You can significantly enhance your message using open gestures and smiles. Speak with conviction, enthusiasm, and passion. To accomplish this, you must speak using open gestures and with a warm smile. Remember, openness equals likeability. Here are three rules for gestures and smiling:

- ► Be aware of nervous gestures and stop them.
- ► Lift the apples of your cheeks—smile.
- ► Feel your smile, but beware: phony smiles don't work.

5. **Concentrate on your voice and vocal variety.** Use intonation and inflection in your voice. Speaking in a monotone can be deadly and can put your listeners to sleep.

   Observe and practice the following rules to add energy to your voice:

   - ► Make your voice naturally authoritative; speak from the diaphragm.
   - ► Put your voice on a roller coaster; practice reading from magazines using intonation and inflection. Watch network news broadcasts to see how the professionals draw you into a story.
   - ► Be aware of your telephone voice; it represents 84 percent of the emotional impact when people can't see you.
   - ► Smile when talking on the telephone; people can feel your smile right through the phone.
   - ► Put your real feelings into your voice.

6. **Energize your words, and avoid using nonwords.** Energize your words and avoid using nonwords that are meaningless and take away from your message. Follow these rules to energize your message:

   - ► Build your vocabulary, especially with synonyms.
   - ► Paint word pictures. Create motion and emotion with metaphors.
   - ► Beware of jargon, especially medical jargon. Say "operating room" instead of "OR."
   - ► Avoid meaningless nonwords, like *ah* and *um*, or words used to stall like, *so*, *well*, and *you know*. Replace those words with a silent pause. A properly timed pause adds drama, energy, and power to your message. Again, listen to the professionals on the network news.

7. **Create listener involvement.** Humans communicate, and books dispense information. Try using the following techniques to add an extra punch to your communication:

   - ► Use a strong opening. Make it visual and energetic by including pauses, action and motion, and joy and laughter.
   - ► Maintain eye communication. When you enter the room for a group interview, survey your listeners for three to five seconds, gauge, and adjust.

▸ Lean toward your listeners.

▸ Create interest by maintaining eye contact and having high energy.

8. **Use humor effectively**. I do not recommend that you tell jokes at your interview, and remember that fun is better than funny. The goal is not comedy but connection. Find the form of humor that works for you, and be natural.

    I hope you can now see why our friend John hasn't gotten accepted to PA school, even though he had excellent credentials on paper. The key to having success at your interview is to have harmony in the verbal, vocal, and visual components of your message.

CHAPTER 10

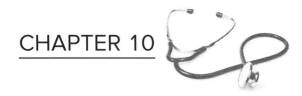

Frequently Asked Questions

Over the years, PA school applicants have asked me many of the same questions. In this chapter I will present some of these questions and provide the answers in a question-and-answer format.

Question 1: Will the admissions committee know what programs I'm applying to?

Debra is applying to ten different PA programs this cycle. Some of them are master's level, some of them are bachelor's level, and one of them is at the associate's level. During her interview, she was asked, "Name all of the programs that you applied to and why you chose those specific programs." She was also asked, "Which program will you choose if you get into multiple programs, and why?"

Debra was a little taken aback by this question. She hadn't thought about the reasoning behind her choices. In fact, she wasn't even sure if she should tell the committee where else she applied. She wasn't sure if they had some way of *knowing*.

Debra decided not to divulge all of the programs that she actually applied to and told the committee, "This program is my number-one choice because of the program's mission statement: 'Working in underserved populations.'"

How well did Debra handle this question?

First of all, many programs do ask this question. Debra should have thought about each and every program she was applying to and what her philosophy was behind making those choices. Many applicants never really stop to think about it. I always ask this question when I do mock interviews with applicants that I coach, and I usually get the same response: "Will they know what programs I'm applying to?"

Does it really matter if they know or not? Every applicant should be honest and have a philosophy for choosing a particular PA program. Some people want to stay in a certain geographical area because they have a family or because they will save money if they can live at home. Some applicants choose programs that are all at the master's level. Others use the technique of choosing a few programs that are "dream" choices—programs they really want to attend but know they fall short in comparison to students who actually get accepted. Then they choose a few programs that are a good fit for their qualifications, programs they would be happy to attend and whose qualifications match those of actual first-year accepted students. Finally, they choose a few schools that are "safety" schools; though these programs are not their first or second choices, they know they exceed the qualifications of actual first-year students. The reality is that most applicants never stop to think about why they are choosing the programs they apply to.

Here are ten common reasons why you might select particular programs:

1. They are in a convenient geographical region. Perhaps you have family or children and you live in close proximity to these programs including a short commuting distance.

2. They offer master's-level programs: you want to earn a master's degree, and you are choosing only PA programs that offer a master's degree.

3. You meet all of the prerequisites and requirements: this is a logical reason for choosing programs. You have the best chance of getting into these schools.

4. You are choosing top-ten or prestigious schools: your goal is to get the best-quality education, irrespective of any of the other reasons.

5. The programs have a good first-time pass/fail rate on the PANCE: you want to be assured that if you invest the time and money into a two-year graduate program, you'll be able to pass the boards and work as a PA.

6. The programs are new: these are the programs that you think will give you the best chance of acceptance. You just want to become a PA, and nothing else matters.

7. You like the focus of the programs: maybe you're interested in a surgical focus, a focus on working in underserved areas, or a religious focus. It would be difficult to explain why you are applying to Cornell, which has a surgical focus, but also to a program with a focus on working in primary care in underserved areas.

8. You've made random choices: if you have no reasoning for choosing the programs you are applying to, it may be difficult to answer the question at the interview.

9. The programs have no requirement for the GRE: I wouldn't disclose this reason to the admissions committee. Try to find another common thread among your choices.

10. The programs have long-standing clinical rotation sites: finding quality clinical-rotation sites is a long process for PA school programs. Acquiring good clinical-rotation sites is a process of trial and error, which can take a few years to refine.

For example, when a new program sends out its first class of students to various clinical-rotation sites, some may report back that the rotation was disappointing. Perhaps the clinical rotation site allows medical students to be the top dogs on the floor or in the operating room (OR). The PA students are assigned all of the menial tasks on the floor, and in the OR they are usually the third assistant, only allowed to hold retractors and usually not able to observe the actual procedure.

The program will then need to look for another clinical rotation site that may be more PA student friendly and one that will provide a better-quality experience. Refining all of the clinical-rotation sites is an ongoing process and a necessary one.

Acquiring excellent clinical opportunities for PA students is important because a lot of what you'll learn on your clinical rotations will be helpful when answering questions on the Physician Assistant National Certification Exam.

Exercise: Is there a common thread among your chosen programs?

Complete this exercise to see if you can find a common thread among the programs that you are choosing. This will help you solidify your answer when asked, "Why have you selected these programs?" I recommend you answer these questions honestly. Maybe you'll find no pattern. Whatever the case may be, you should be ready to answer this question at your interview, and completing and reviewing this exercise will provide you with the insight you need to come with an educated response.

Program	Reason for Applying Here

Now ask yourself, what is the common denominator in your choice of these particular programs?

_____

_____

_____

_____

_____

Question 2: Is shadowing or volunteering considered health care experience?

There are six categories of "experience" relative to an application for PA school. Check the websites of the programs you apply to and look under the requirements section to see the exact type of experience required. Most programs do not count volunteer experience as health care experience hours.

EXPERIENCE CATEGORIES

In this section you should enter your professional experiences in each of the following categories:

Patient-Care Experience

Experiences in which you are directly responsible for a patient's care—for example, prescribing medication, performing procedures, directing a course of treatment, working on patients as an active nurse or EMT, etc.

1. _____ Hours accumulated: _____

2. _____ Hours accumulated: _____

3. _____ Hours accumulated: _____

4. _____ Hours accumulated: _____

5. _____ Hours accumulated: _____

Total hours: _____

Health-Care Experience

Both paid and unpaid work in a health or a health-related field where you are not directly responsible for a patient's care—for example, filling prescriptions, performing clerical work, delivering patient food, cleaning patient rooms, working as a scribe or hospital volunteer, etc.

1. _____ Hours accumulated: _____
2. _____ Hours accumulated: _____
3. _____ Hours accumulated: _____
4. _____ Hours accumulated: _____
5. _____ Hours accumulated: _____

Total hours: _____

Employment

Paid work done outside of the health-care field, such as a retail or restaurant job.

1. _____ Hours accumulated: _____
2. _____ Hours accumulated: _____
3. _____ Hours accumulated: _____
4. _____ Hours accumulated: _____
5. _____ Hours accumulated: _____

Total hours: _____

Shadowing

Time spent officially following and observing a health-care professional at work, preferably a physician assistant.

1. _____ Hours accumulated: _____
2. _____ Hours accumulated: _____
3. _____ Hours accumulated: _____
4. _____ Hours accumulated: _____
5. _____ Hours accumulated: _____

Total hours: _____

Research

Research projects done in addition to classroom work; research should *not* appear as credit on a school transcript.

1. _____ Hours accumulated: _____
2. _____ Hours accumulated: _____
3. _____ Hours accumulated: _____
4. _____ Hours accumulated: _____
5. _____ Hours accumulated: _____

Total hours: _____

Volunteer

Volunteer work done outside of the health-care field—for example, working for Habitat for Humanity, tutoring students, participating in or working for a fundraiser walk or blood drive, etc.

1. _____ Hours accumulated: _____
2. _____ Hours accumulated: _____
3. _____ Hours accumulated: _____
4. _____ Hours accumulated: _____
5. _____ Hours accumulated: _____

Total hours: _____

Question 3: Do I have a chance?

Amy would like to know what her chances are of getting into PA school. She has a 3.5 overall GPA and a 3.65 GPA in the sciences. Amy has twenty-five hundred hours of medical experience as a paramedic, and fifteen hundred volunteer hours with the local hospital. She meets all of the prerequisites of the programs that she is applying to, and she also has three hundred hours of shadowing experience with PAs in family practice, cardiology, and general surgery.

The question behind the question in this example is, do you think Amy will get *accepted* to a PA program? On paper Amy has great credentials; however, getting accepted to a PA program involves more than just meeting or exceeding the prerequisites.

Given Amy's qualifications, one would think Amy has a strong chance of getting into PA school. However, if Amy writes a poor essay, her chances are less than likely that she will be invited for an interview. Therefore, her chances of acceptance are slim to none.

If Amy makes it to the interview but fails to make an emotional connection with the admissions committee, her chances are practically zero.

The bottom line is that this question cannot be answered. I would tell Amy that she has great qualifications, but that's all I can offer. I've personally interviewed applicants who looked great on paper but interviewed horribly. Applicants who use my mock interview services quickly learn that they need to do a lot of work in order to claim their seat in the upcoming class.

Question 4: How do I improve my chances of getting accepted?

Following the list below will help improve your chances.

1. Meet or exceed *all* of the program's requirements and prerequisite classes.

2. Continue to gain health-care experience right up until the time you interview.

3. Join the American Academy of Physician Assistants and your state or constituent chapter of the AAPA. Doing this will allow you access to a constant stream of information for and about PAs at the state and national level. Joining these organizations shows passion and motivation and will help you tremendously at the interview.

4. Write and rewrite several drafts of your essay before submitting it to CASPA. Capture the attention of the reader in the first paragraph by using a vignette or telling a story. Be sure there are no spelling or grammatical errors, and be sure that it flows well and creates interest. Using vignettes will captivate the reader. Discuss your soft skills and avoid clichéd statements like "I've always wanted to help people." Finally, *answer the question being asked*. If you read your essay and it doesn't specifically address why you want to become a PA (not why you want to work in health care), you need to do it over.

   Remember, the essay is your ticket to the interview, and if you do a poor job writing it, you have no chance of being accepted. If you need help with your essay, utilize my essay edit and review services, which can be found on my website, andrewrodican.com.

5. Attend the program's open house. This is a great opportunity to learn more about what the program is looking for in strong applicants and also to learn the mission and values of the program. Additionally, you'll have

the opportunity to meet faculty and students. The faculty will remember you at the interview and probably score you a bit higher for taking the time to visit the school. Attending the open house will go a long way to show your motivation.

6. Talk to as many students as you can, and find out what they value most in the program. Their answers to your questions will go a long way in helping you answer the interview question, "Why are you selecting our program?"

Question 5: How can I best prepare for the interview?

Remember this simple fact: *failing to prepare is preparing to fail*. In this book I've introduced you to the various interview-question types and advised how to answer them. Be sure to read my book *How to "Ace" the Physician Assistant School Interview*, which provides the questions and answers to the most common PA school interview questions. Also, I strongly suggest taking advantage of my mock-interview services. I will not only ask you the questions you need to know, I will critique you along the way, advise you on your presentation and how to improve your answers, and teach you how to make an emotional connection. I guarantee that you will feel much less anxious and much more prepared after completing these services.

Additionally, do your homework on the program itself. Review every page of the program's website. Here are some things you must absolutely know before interviewing:

1. What year did the program start?

2. What is the school's first-time pass/fail rate on the boards over the past five years?

3. Does the program have a cadaver lab?

4. Who teaches the classes—PAs, physicians, researchers, or fellows pursuing specialty certification in their chosen specialty? Fellows are MDs who have recently completed a residency program and are pursuing board certification in a specialty, like cardiology, endocrinology, surgery, etc. If you think about it, fellows have the most current knowledge base in their specialty and have a lot of passion for that specialty. In my opinion, you will learn the most up-to-date information from fellows.

5. Are the rotation sites well established?

6. What are the options for clinical rotations in terms of diversity, international rotations, and elective rotations?

7. What is the mission of the program? Are there any notable features about the program? (See appendix.)

8. Learn about the program faculty who may be interviewing you: Are they involved with PA politics at the state or national level? Have they received any awards? How long have they been on the program's faculty?

Question 6: How do I find PAs to shadow?

There are several ways to find PAs to shadow. Obviously, the easiest way is to ask any PAs that you work with or who you know personally. Another way is to actually call or e-mail PAs working at local clinics and ask if they would allow you to shadow them. Call a local PA program and ask them for suggestions. Join your state chapter of the AAPA, attend some meetings, and contact the chapter's president for a list of PAs who are willing to allow applicants to shadow them. Many of the state chapters will have a list of PAs who agree to allow shadowing at their places of work.

Question 7: How many programs should I apply to?

In my opinion, applicants should apply to at least five programs in order to demonstrate motivation for becoming a PA and to increase their chances of getting accepted. If you apply to only one program, you are putting all your eggs in one basket. Admissions committees may think that perhaps you're just testing the water.

If your goal is to become a PA, and not just to get into a particular program, I would recommend that you choose one or two dream programs (your first choices). They may even be a bit of a stretch based on your credentials, but it's worth the effort to apply anyway.

Next, select a couple of competitive, established programs for which you are a good fit. These might not be your dream programs but would nevertheless offer a quality education.

Finally, select one or two safety programs—programs where you'll be a strong applicant and you would consider attending if accepted.

Question 8: Should I still apply to PA school if I am short one prerequisite?

If you look on the websites of most programs, they will answer this question for you. The website may point out that you must have all of the prerequisites accomplished by a certain deadline.

To put this question into another perspective, you should consider how competitive it is to get into PA school. Most programs receive hundreds of qualified applicants who meet all of the requirements. Why would they consider an applicant who has not met all of the prerequisites?

Question 9: If I don't get accepted to one of my dream programs but get accepted elsewhere, should I wait another year to apply to my dream programs a second time or accept the offer from the program that accepted me?

You know the old saying, "A bird in the hand is worth two in the bush." I would recommend that you consider the school's first-time pass/fail rate, and if it's competitive, accept the offer and fulfill your goal of becoming a PA. The only reason I might suggest waiting another year is if the program that accepts you is not yet fully accredited or is in its first year. Even then, there still is no guarantee that you will get accepted to your dream programs the next year.

Question 10: Should I send a thank-you letter after I interview?

PA school applicants commonly ask this question. In my experience on admissions committees, your fate is determined way before you'll even have the time to send a thank-you letter. I never sent one thank-you letter, and I got accepted to all of the programs I applied to. On the other hand, sending a letter certainly won't hurt, but it may not be necessary or improve your chances of acceptance.

FINAL THOUGHTS

When I made my decision to apply to PA school, I was thirty-four years old, married, with two small children, and I had a great job in sales, earning more money than I was going to make as a new PA. I would be lying if I didn't admit that I initially had some reservations about making the leap into a new career field and having to borrow thousands of dollars for PA school. However, I had wanted to be a PA since leaving the navy after serving for four years as a navy corpsman. I distinctly remember thinking, *I don't want to look back when I'm forty and wonder, what if?* I made the decision and never looked back.

My investment paid off more than I could have imagined. I've had the opportunity to work in a variety of clinical settings: cardiothoracic surgery, occupational medicine, cardiology, bariatric medicine (in which I owned my own practice for eight years), and currently family practice. I continue to live a life well beyond my wildest dreams.

As you begin your journey on your PAth to PA school, I urge you to focus on your goal and never look back. I promise you will not regret your decision.

I know this for a fact because I've had the honor of helping thousands of PA school applicants achieve success since 1997, and I want to help you too.

If you meet the qualifications and prerequisites of the PA programs you wish to attend, and you read, digest, and follow the recommendations presented in this workbook, you'll be well on your way to success. Additionally, if you invest your time in completing the exercises in this book, you will be far ahead of the competition.

Remember, a journey of a thousand miles begins with a single step. Commit your goal to writing, begin prioritizing your objectives, and follow your dream, never looking back.

I wish you the best of luck in your pursuit of becoming a PA-C, and I look forward to meeting you as a colleague one day.

APPENDIX

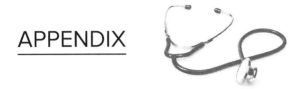

Forty Sample Essays

In this section, you will find sample essays from others who have gone through this process. All of the writers of these essays were asked to interview for at least one school of their choice.

These essays are meant to assist you by giving you examples from which to learn. You may like aspects of some essays and not like aspects of others. Some have errors—grammatical and otherwise—so see if you can catch those and then recognize how easy it is to submit an essay with errors.

Plagiarizing from these essays is illegal. As I said, they are provided for you as tools which you can use to learn to write a quality essay.

Essay 1 (826 words)

"Your wife is dying!" Hearing those words marked a turning point in my life. When it came time for the birth of our fourth son, financial circumstances found us without medical insurance. However, with three previously healthy deliveries, we believed a home birth with a mid-wife would be okay. The birth went great until my wife had a retained placenta. In my ignorance I calmly held my wife in my arms as she was slowly bleeding to death. When the mid-wife finally alerted us to the true nature of our situation, I hit a point of fear and desperation I had never known before. I was powerless to help my wife except to race her to the hospital where a very capable physician and staff were able to calmly administer three units of blood and confidently perform the necessary lifesaving procedures. Although life pursuits had initially taken me through other vocations, this experience became the catalyst for our family decision for me to become a Physician Assistant (PA).

Entering the world of the PA is an incredible challenge. I have overcome other incredible challenges before, especially when I walked onto the men's gymnastics team as a freshman in college. Because my last gymnastics class was in elementary school, I lacked the basic training and experience of my teammates. Yet, what I lacked in preparation I made up for with passion and dedication. I did not compete as a gymnast my first year on the team but I was determined to succeed. The following years I did compete as a part of our championship team and was the team captain my senior year. Like my experience with the gymnastic team, I am confident that I can handle the rigors, work ethic, and commitment required to become a champion PA.

Being a part of the community and helping others thrive has always been a driving force in my life. Growing up on the Navajo Indian Reservation there were ample opportunities to serve. Organizing church and Boy Scout service projects designed to improve our community were regular activities for me. Formally and informally, I tutored friends and peers in high school and college. Later, as a real estate agent, I found great joy and satisfaction in helping families find their way to owning their first homes. As I did in the Upward Bound programs of my high school, I have always worked to help members of my community improve their circumstances and strive for better things in life.

Being a PA is the best way to focus my desire to improve and help my community in a meaningful way with my passion for excellence. When I was growing up on the Reservation, there was only a two-room clinic with a rotating doctor and receptionist. Frequently, we traveled hours just to get into a town with a fully staffed clinic and modern healthcare facilities and equipment. Being a PA would make it possible to take full-time help back to the reservation and to other towns in similar situations. So many of my friends deal with chronic pains and problems that may have been prevented with current medical care. As a PA, I will have the training to help care for my friends, family, and community, and to break the poor health cycle by helping their children have a better quality of life.

Once my family and I realized that becoming a PA was the route I should take, we took immediate action. I quit my job and returned to school full-time to take the PA program pre-requisite coursework as quickly as possible. I also took the time to acquire patient care experience. My patient care experience has been an opportunity to work with mentally ill patients—a significant population of medically underserved people right here in our communities. Because of my driving desire to help, I have frequently been with my patients six and seven days a week often volunteering to stay late, picking up extra shifts, and working on all of the units in the hospital. It has been satisfying and fulfilling for me to see so many of my patients go from their deepest problems to developing a significant measure of mental health and control and being discharged from the hospital to return to society.

The exciting and challenging world of a healthcare provider and the rewarding career as a Physician Assistant is about being able to care for people, especially the underserved members of our community. I want to spend my life caring for people who really need and deserve quality healthcare. Once trained, I will be able to take my medical experience back to the Reservation, and to other deserving communities a well. While my life has taken some interesting turns, I am someone who is prepared for the academic rigors, the strict work ethic, the compassion for patients, and the caring to reach out to our community that makes for a truly great PA.

Essay 2 (940 words)

Early on June 25, 2011, as Flight 3906 began its ascent, my seatmate grabbed my arm. "There's something wrong with that boy," she warned. "I think he may be having an anxiety attack." In the seat behind me, Garrett, sweat running down his face, leaned forward and clutched his abdomen. Calling on my training as an EMT and a technician in Yale-New Haven Hospital's Emergency Department, and remembering countless conversations with my husband, an ED physician, I did a quick assessment and gathered a history. This 16-year-old was very sick, and when the plane reached altitude minutes later, Garrett's pulse became rapid and irregular.

I told the flight attendant that Garrett needed emergency medical attention, and an RN came forward to help. I reported my findings to the nurse, who assumed control of communication with the flight crew. When Garrett was no longer able to sit upright, we lay him on the cabin floor and swabbed his face with wet towels, but his pain was relentless. His lips were white and his pupils dilated; at times he became verbally unresponsive. When we finally reached the Charlotte airport, no ambulance or emergency team awaited us.

After we landed, the RN walked away from the patient, and first responders rebuffed my efforts to communicate with them, so I also walked away and hurried to catch my next flight. That night, Garrett died.

Months later, I sat in a stuffy conference room, responding to questions from a US Airways investigator. After two hours of questioning, her tone changed, her voice hardened, and she asked suspiciously, "Why did you call his parents?" I stared at the red light on the tape recorder and tried to compose my thoughts. It occurred to me that she thought I might be looking for compensation. "My brother was killed when he was 18," I said. "I've seen what happens to parents when their children die. They have questions. Most of all, they ask, 'When my child was suffering, did anyone help him? When he was in pain, was there someone with him who cared?'"

Had I been in that situation a few years earlier, I would have wanted to help, but with no training, I would have held back. I probably would not have realized how sick he really was.

Just a few years before that flight, I had been a public relations executive, helping to grow a business from $6 million to $70 million in five years. I worked hard and was good at my job, but I felt no passion for it. For emotional fulfillment, I looked outside my job. I volunteered on political campaigns, assisted

with communication efforts to fight my neighborhood's epidemic of teen sui-
cide, and tutored inner-city students. All of this ended in catastrophe. In 2006,
my company restructured, and I lost my highpaying job. My house flooded. I
became very ill, and my oncologist performed surgery. Two days later, I hemor-
rhaged and received last rites and additional emergency surgery. My father, who
was brilliant, funny, and the rock of my life, died.

Stripped of all pretense, income, and power, I was completely humbled,
but it was oddly liberating. Suddenly, I was free to question the trajectory of my
life, and I wondered how I had strayed so far from my ideals. I didn't know how
I could find my way back. By coincidence, I heard of an EMT training program
at Northeastern University. I enrolled, passed the entrance exam, applied to
and entered nursing school. I fought hard for a job as an ED Tech at Yale-New
Haven Hospital, and I secured that position.

At YNHH, I discovered many things about myself and realized I had a
talent for spotting the very sick. Having suffered the indignities of failure, poor
judgment, illness, and powerlessness, I had developed genuine compassion for
the poor and the disenfranchised. I sat for hours with mentally ill, alcoholic,
and addicted patients. I held their hands and sometimes endured their angry
insults. I bandaged wounds and dried tears. I cleaned up blood and excrement.
I made mistakes and learned from them. To paraphrase Martin Luther King, I
felt the arc of my own moral universe bending slowly toward justice.

At Yale-New Haven Hospital, I was part of a team of dedicated and excep-
tionally capable people, from physicians to nurses, technicians, and physician
assistants. I became intrigued by the work of PAs and the integration of the physician's practice with that of the PA. I learned about the differential diagnosis
model and its contrast with the nursing diagnosis paradigm that I continued to
find so alien. I believed my choices were limited because I had made mistakes
in college and had not wanted to endure the sacrifice of medical school and
residency. Although I was already in nursing school when I worked at YNHH,
I began to formulate plans for becoming a PA. When my husband and I moved
to Kentucky, I enrolled in pre-requisite classes for PA programs.

Some have questioned why I would take on the burdens of a PA career
at an age when others are seeking freedom and leisure. In response, I think of
the words of author David Foster Wallace: "Of course there are all different
kinds of freedom," he said, "and the kind that is most precious you will not hear
much talked about in the great outside world of winning, achieving, and dis-
playing. The really important kind of freedom involves attention, awareness,
discipline, and effort, and being truly able to care about other people and to
sacrifice for them, over and over, in myriad, petty, unsexy ways, every day. That
is real freedom."

Essay 3 (671 words)

The dictionary defines cancer as a malignant growth that spreads destructively, yet after my diagnosis with thyroid cancer in 2008 and subsequent treatment and recuperation, I made a positive discovery. It was through my experience with radiation therapy that I first encountered the physician assistant profession. Growing up in rural Wyoming, my only exposure to healthcare was the traditional physician-and-nurse model. My experience as a cancer patient was the first time a practitioner other than a physician was partially responsible for my treatment. My consultation with the PA was very thorough; he took the time to get to know me on a personal level and developed a connection with me prior to my meeting with the doctor. While highly educated and professional, the physician did not have the same rapport with me that the PA had developed. The PA took the time to make me feel comfortable with him, helped me understand my scheduled treatment, and explained the process of healing following my treatment.

I am fascinated by the functions of the healthy human body as well as its healing capacity when recovering from injury, disease, neglect, or abuse; the human body and spirit are truly miraculous healers. I have been interested in science and medicine since high school when my mother was attending nursing school and having me quiz her in preparation for her upcoming exams. From that point on, I knew I wanted a career in medicine. Enrolled in college, I followed a pre-professional track that culminated with a degree in Kinesiology and Health Promotion.

After graduating from the University of Wyoming, I traveled, gained new experiences, and found a job working in occupational health. Although I enjoyed it, I worked alone and traveled to a new site every couple of days. This was a lonely experience and did not provide the opportunity to build new relationships or foster old ones, so I changed jobs and took a position as a personal fitness instructor. I had a variety of clients, each with their own needs and expectations; some were rehabilitating from an injury, some were working to prevent injury, and others wanted to improve their health and fitness. I learned a great deal and enjoyed working one-on-one with individuals to address their problems and help improve their lives. Although this was an enjoyable experience, I felt it was still not the right fit for me.

In 2008, I took the opportunity to work at a pediatric dental office. During my time there, I was fortunate to work directly with patients on a daily basis. This afforded me the opportunity to get to know the patients as more than simply "the crown in room 2" or "the cleaning in room 5," as I had heard the staff refer to them. I became acquainted with them on a personal level, developed a rapport, and helped them through their procedures. One patient in particular was terrified of getting an injection, and I was able to keep her calm and comfort her during the procedure; now she is no longer terrified of the dentist and requests my presence at her visits. Empathizing with a patient during a difficult time means a great deal to me as a healthcare provider, and this motivates me to pursue a career as a PA.

The most important issues for patients are to feel they have been heard and to know their concerns have been addressed; four years of patient and client interaction have enabled me to become an excellent listener. Using this skill, I have found that patients will provide necessary information while developing a positive relationship with their healthcare provider. Having a flexible career in the healthcare field with multiple opportunities for service is what motivates me establish a career as a PA. My goal is to work in a rural location where I can build a practice, raise my family, and become an active member of my community. I am confident I will be an excellent PA and will always be grateful for this opportunity.

Essay 4 (751 words)

180 degrees:

The Academy Awards for advertising was a black-tie gala event held in Washington, D.C. I held three gold "Addys" in my right hand and two silver ones in my left, yet I had never felt so unfulfilled in my life. As I recalled the goal I had set twenty-three years earlier, to pursue a medical career, I saw that event as my personal tipping point.

0 degrees:

As an Airman at the David Grant Medical Center, the combination of working closely with administrators and medical staff while attending to patients provided me with an excellent introduction to healthcare. Observing the dynamics of hospital administration allowed me to experience the politics, ethics, and multidisciplinary team functions of the medical and support staff. In an organization that discourages fraternization between officers and enlisted personnel, the work of physician assistants (PA) resonated with me. The PAs seemed to connect with both groups while earning the respect and admiration of staff and patients, and this is something I had personally experienced from the perspective of a patient. As an anxious eighteen-year-old inpatient, a PA treated my injury and reassured me I would not be disciplined for the situation that had caused it. I never forgot how he took the time to listen, empathize, and make me laugh about my circumstances.

90 degrees:

While working at Danbury Hospital after leaving the Air Force, I focused on a degree in Hospital Administration, but a mentor convinced me to pursue a career in marketing. As a Grey Advertising account executive (AE), I expanded my leadership and soft skills. As the liaison between agency and client, I managed multiple projects from inception to completion in stressful, high-pressure, time-sensitive situations. I also became adept at translating and presenting an idea or strategy to clients, and I found myself naturally comfortable when working with senior executives and diverse teammates. I enjoyed leading and participating in teams and working with interesting individuals who possessed a broad assortment of skills while, together, we produced great products for our clients and achieved agency goals.

270 degrees:

After thirteen years in advertising, I yearned for a career that would allow me to become deeply involved with individual wellness and healthcare. Changing my career will only make sense if my past work experiences and skills can be utilized in the transition. Every AE knows that, to become successful, one must be multifaceted and able to anticipate the needs of the client. This philosophy parallels a PA's role as a healthcare provider and has prepared me for the PA profession. My return to medicine began with sacrificing a steady salary, attending college, working as an EMT, and volunteering as a physical therapist's aide, a nurse's aide, and a patient advocate/medical assistant at Shepherd's Clinic. Maintaining many regular PA follows, subscribing to PA journals, joining PA organizations, and continuing to read numerous PA-related books, such as A Kernel in the Pod, has reinforced my determination to join this profession.

I have always enjoyed giving back to my community, but volunteering at Shepherd's Clinic changed my life. Working with PAs and patients in a near-universal healthcare environment has been rewarding and fulfilling, and it has inspired me to use my education and work experience to provide the highest quality of healthcare. In the Air Force, no one has to pay for medical treatment, and the clinic provides free clinical and wellness care for indigenous and underserved patients. During my first PA follow, I met a gentleman named Jimmy during his first visit to the clinic. Jimmy had been released from prison after serving thirteen years and required a battery of tests and treatments. He now calls regularly and specifically asks for me, hoping to learn more about the clinic's latest wellness programs or just have a quick chat. Jimmy has kept his promises to maintain his therapy, find employment, and live his life as an integral part of the community.

360 degrees:

Someone told me that my life has now come full circle. Just as Jimmy resumed his life with a new passion for well-being, my passion, as a PA, is to help others achieve good health and wellness. As a PA student, I will challenge myself to produce the equivalent of five Addys for each patient and for the PA profession. Adding PA skills to my leadership and administrative experience will provide an excellent foundation for the achievement of my long-term goal of creating and practicing in primary care facilities similar to the Shepherd's Clinic.

Essay 5 (754 words)

Sir Winston Churchill once said, "We make a living by what we get; we make a life by what we give." Without knowing it, the sentiment of this quote has guided me throughout my adult life towards what I feel is my destiny: to become a physician assistant. I first felt this inner drive as a high school teenager with an interest in veterinary medicine, which prompted me to volunteer at local animal hospitals. There I developed the skill of providing thoughtful medical attention to patients who could not convey their symptoms with words. The level of empathy, compassion, and patience required to work with animals has stayed with me, and it is at the core of my patient care skills today. This same energy made itself known once again as a young adult in college; when many of my peers were involved in social activism, I joined them but decided that I could be of best service as a street medic. I quickly developed skills in treating people using the limited means I had available. The level of focus, drive, and quick-thinking necessary to assist the injured inspired and motivated me. I wanted more.

At the completion of a course in wilderness survival first aid, I was offered the opportunity to teach the course. My instructor always told me that teaching is learning twice, which I took to heart. I became a certified instructor and not only taught the course to mountaineers but also taught CPR to various organizations and school groups, taught marine safety survival to coworkers and fellow mariners, and developed a Spanish CPR curriculum for the Latino community in my district. I continue teaching today, having developed a strong passion for sharing medical and survival information.

After earning my undergraduate degree in zoology I pursued a career as a fisheries biologist, and for the past 15 years I have been involved in extended field research projects in the Bering Sea and Gulf of Alaska. Long hours, harsh conditions, and intricate scientific research challenge the best people when working on a ship. As a crew leader for the past 12 years I understand that everyone's lives depend on each other when at sea; thus, effective leadership, positive teamwork and a little humor are essential to completing the tasks while maintaining morale and retuning home safely. These life skills are applicable far beyond the ocean.

Seven years ago I felt yet another pull to be of service and became a part-time fire fighter EMT. In this role, I find that patient care continues to be the most intriguing aspect of the job. We are given the trust to enter people's homes, to have their personal lives revealed and to effectively make quick medical assessments while providing comfort and reassurance. The only frustration in the pre-hospital emergency setting is the limited diagnostic tools and treatment options available to us, and often I find myself wishing we could do more for our patients. Our patient contact ends when we transfer care to the emergency room staff, leaving me curious as to the outcome of our initial treatment and what, if anything, we could have done to help more.

In 2010, I participated in a medical relief project in Guatemala. As a Latina born in Chile and fluent in Spanish, my initial tasks were to assist in translation between the patients and doctors. However, as the clinic became more hectic it was clear that I could and should do more. I used my EMT skills to quickly triage the patients and perform more in-depth initial assessments ahead of the doctors, which increased our efficiency. The day the lead physician asked me, "Have you ever considered a career as a PA?" was the day that changed my life. I began to learn everything about the profession, and having now thoroughly explored the physician assistant career and having gained valuable knowledge from my various PA job shadows, it is clear to me that this is the career I want for the rest of my life.

I am eager to bring the skills I have gathered from all aspects of my life to the PA profession and I look forward to being part of a medical team in a collaborative environment between doctors, nurses, and other PAs contributing to the ultimate goal of effective health care for our patients. I eagerly await the challenges and rewards of this career and know that I will gain tremendous personal satisfaction from having given the best care possible to my patients.

Essay 6 (393 words)

I'm in the middle of an open field of alfalfa hay. The sweet smell of honeysuckle in the air relaxes me as I ride on the green John Deere. To my left, the hay has been raked in single file rows, ready to be baled. To my right is a blanket of hay needing to be raked in a line before the hot July sun dries it out. My father calls to me from the field entrance as he unhooks the gate to pull his blue Ford tractor and baler through. There is more to do. Each summer my dad and I each spend about 300 hours on tractors baling hay for our cattle in preparation for the snowy winter months, a common activity for people in my community. I adore my small hometown, and my dream is to return there to fulfill my other passion—to serve my community as a healthcare provider.

Working on a beef farm has always fed my soul. I shadowed a large animal veterinarian, thinking that veterinary medicine might the right path for me, but the veterinarian cautioned me against the field if I wanted to raise a family because I would be on call day and night. Though taking care of animals appeals to my nurturing spirit, this experience shifted my focus to a deeper interest in taking care of people, which brought healthcare to my attention as a career. While in high school, I shadowed a pharmacist at Wytheville Community Hospital, thinking pharmacy might be a satisfying career. I pursued pharmacology until my sophomore year in college, when my experience at the University of Virginia Outpatient Pharmacy showed me that spending all day at a counter filling prescriptions and helping the pharmacist was simply too monotonous and isolated for me.

A light bulb went off one day as I was speaking with my best friend. I shared with her that I was having second thoughts about pharmacy and that I craved more interaction with people. She asked if I had considered going to med school, but I had a litany of reasons why that was not for me, including the length of time it takes to finally be able to practice, the enormous debt I would accrue, and the liability doctors are burdened with. She said, "Why not be a physician assistant?" Though I hate to admit it, that was the first time I had even heard of the role, so I starting doing my research. I explored the undergraduate Physician Assistant Club at the University of Virginia, and soon fell in love with the idea of becoming a PA. At one club meeting, a speaker from a PA program explained how physician assistants work autonomously yet collaboratively with physicians. He highlighted the versatility of the career, and described how PAs are in high demand, particularly in rural areas. Like a bolt of lightening, it struck me that this was the perfect path for me. I began shadowing a family physician assistant in my hometown, who spoke about the opportunities and challenges of being a physician assistant. I loved the fact that she had direct patient interaction while being able to refer questions to a physician when she needed further opinions. I knew that this balance of independence and collaboration suited my personality to a tee, but it was a personal encounter with healthcare that cemented my passion for the profession.

Three months ago, a close friend of mine was diagnosed with Squamous-Cell Carcinoma, a shock to his family and friends. He was thrown into a blur of appointments for surgery, radiation, and chemotherapy. Worried about his potential for survival, he and his wife and son were left with no choice but to put their faith in the healthcare staff—from physicians to PAs to nurses— to save his life. I saw the difference made by the bedside manner of those caring for him, both positive and negative, and because even more passionate about establishing a caring, empathetic, and devoted patient-physician and family-physician relationship. For patients to put their trust in my hands will be a tremendous honor that will give me a tremendous sense of purpose each day.

My goal is to practice as a physician assistant in my rural hometown in Southwest Virginia, building trusting patient-physician relationships and impacting the overall health of my community. As I drive by the lines of fields on my way to work as a PA, the sweet scent of alfalfa and honeysuckle will reassure me that I am right where I am supposed to be.

Essay 7 (500 words)

The wide-ranging experiences of nearly losing my father, volunteering, teaching middle-schoolers and running have led to my wholehearted pursuit of a career as a physician assistant.

The most powerful experience of my life was when my father was mistreated for Lyme disease, suffered a subdural hematoma, and underwent emergency brain surgery. We were told that his odds were long, but I thank God and the medical team for his full recovery. Above any other, this experience called me to action and motivated me to pursue a career as a physician assistant where I hope to provide the kind of quality care that my dad received.

My interest in healthcare and helping others was brewing long before my father's illness, however, and I was raised to work hard in pursuit of my passions. In middle school and high school, I volunteered at a hospital and nursing home where I relished my interactions with patients as I provided basic care observed the skilled physician assistants. Though I obviously lacked the technical skills to provide more direct patient care, I learned to build relationships with patients and work alongside medical staff. In college, I directly cared for patients as a personal care attendant and I was hooked; I wanted to utilize my skills to the greatest impact.

Given my passion for new experiences, after college I chose a challenging new path. Armed with only confidence, I took a two-year position as a middle school teacher in a low-income school where I taught teenagers about their bodies, encouraged budding scientists, and led my students and the science department to success. Surprisingly, it was through this experience that I discovered a new angle on my passion for medicine; witnessing the lack of healthcare available to these low-income families was my calling to effect change in the medical field. This two-year teaching commitment gave me a deep understanding of the obstacles of the underprivileged and taught me how to educate a reluctant audience while persevering against challenges.

My classroom work was largely external, but in an internal way, my passion for running has impacted my outlook and my attitude on personal health and preventative care. Through college track and running everything from 5k's to marathons, I'm fascinated by the human body. My pursuit of running and wellness has led me to work with friends and family on their personal fitness goals, which has fed my inquisitiveness about the body while improving my ability to educate others on preventative health and wellness. While internal motivation is critical, to gain more direct clinical experience I am now an emergency room volunteer where I observe staff making make decisions under extreme stress. This exposure only furthered my desire to pursue a career as a physician assistant.

My journey to pursuing my physician assistant degree has involved events and experiences that have given me tremendous appreciation for the role that PA's play in the healthcare continuum. I look forward to taking the next step in this journey to serve others.

Essay 8 (774 words)

"A 73-year-old Caucasian male is brought to the Emergency Room. He appears weak and lethargic. His family members state that they found him in this condition in his apartment and that he has likely not been eating or drinking much over the past two days. What are the patient's principal problems? How would you proceed to treat this patient?"

This is the clinical case that was presented to us during the first day of the Human Pathophysiology and Translational Science (HPTM) PhD program at the University of Texas Medical Branch (UTMB) in September 2011. The graduate program trains scientists to communicate effectively with clinicians and to accelerate the application of basic science discovery from "bench to bedside". This program gave me a special opportunity to join medical students in their courses and clinical encounters for the first six months, focusing primarily on scientific laboratory-based research.

My interest in becoming a physician assistant began in 2010 when I saw a PA for a skin infection. Because of my curiosity about his role, he invited me to observe him for several days; I was impressed by the time he took with patients and the outstanding care he provided, and I was instantly drawn to patient care. As I was completing my master's degree in biomedical science, I gained more direct experience with patients by shadowing more PAs and volunteering in hospitals and community centers. I applied to several PA programs that same year, but unfortunately did not receive an acceptance offer. I was crestfallen and unsure whether to re-apply immediately to PA schools or to continue with a PhD program. Ultimately, I enrolled in UTMB's HPTM PhD program because of the inclusion of clinical work in its curriculum.

Our first courses were gross anatomy and radiology, and by the second week we had dissected the thorax, including the anterior chest wall and breast, pleural cavity and lungs, heart and great vessels. The complexity of the human body fascinated me and I was absolutely hooked. We learned how to identify pathology found on human cadavers, learned to read X-rays and computed tomography scans, bone scans and magnetic resonance imaging to better understand the pathophysiology of diseases. In Problem-Based Learning (PBL) classes, being part of a team that analyzed clinical cases to properly diagnose patients improved my critical thinking skills and taught me how to formulate relevant questions. The intensity and fast pace of the classes was sometimes overwhelming, but strong study skills helped me succeed and enjoy six months of medical school. Moreover, I have had the privilege to observe and scrub in for surgical procedures including mastectomy and removal of liposarcoma. In addition to the PBL classes, the opportunity to join Dr. Chao in her weekly oncological conferences and to listen to doctors across various specialties discuss complicated cases deepened my knowledge and sharpened my problem solving skills.

Though I gained a great deal from this experience, what I enjoyed most was working in a collaborative and high-energy environment, as well as having direct contact with patients—opportunities that simply do not exist inside a scientific laboratory. Thus, I withdrew from the PhD program to pursue a career about which I am truly passionate: becoming a physician assistant. I immediately began shadowing more PAs, I joined the American Academy of Physician Assistants and the Texas Academy of Physician Assistants, and volunteered with the Ronald McDonald House to care for critically ill children. Observing Mr. Celis, a surgical PA at Shriners Burns Hospital, also helped me better understand the aspects of the profession. I was impressed by his autonomy in seeing patients for pre- and post-operative care and in performing minor surgeries. I have also witnessed great PA-physician teamwork through watching a coronary artery bypass surgery operated by Mr. Bratovich, a cardiothoracic surgical PA, with the attending surgeon at the Methodist Hospital in Houston Medical Center. In addition to my clinical exposure to the work of PA's, reading the Journal of the American Academy of Physician Assistants keeps me current about the profession's news and topics. Additionally, I am taking a physiology course and will soon be enrolling in a medical Spanish class.

These experiences have only deepened my desire to pursue a physician assistant career. Since I first applied to PA programs I am more mature, focused, determined and motivated to succeed in an intense curriculum. I wish to integrate and utilize my scientific training and medical background to excel as a student and to become an outstanding healthcare provider. Trained in your rigorous program, I look forward to ultimately becoming a compassionate physician assistant who makes a true difference in the lives of my patients.

Essay 9 (706 words)

My first encounter with a PA occurred during an EMT course as a senior in high school. The clinical rotation required for the course provided me with a fascinating look into a world I wanted to be a part of. I remember being not only impressed, but also inspired by the story of a PA named Jim. He had been a Navy Corpsman assigned to a Marine unit in Vietnam. He explained how his military training and experience had translated into a rewarding career in the civilian world as a PA and what a great fit it was for his personality and medical groundwork. When he described his scope of practice and skill set, I knew then and there that was going to be my goal. I would use Jim's example as a template for my own career. My vocational path is not identical to Jim's, but my entire adult life has been dedicated to working in healthcare

The first step for me was enlisting in the Air Force upon graduation from high school. Early in my career, I was trained as an Independent Duty Medical Technician (IDMT). Although the scope of practice of an IDMT and a PA are vastly different, there is one important similarity—IDMTs are trained to work autonomously in austere conditions under the guidance of a physician. This methodology simultaneously promotes independent practice and a team concept.

As an example of this concept in action, I was deployed as the senior medic for a 90-person construction project in the island nation of St. Kitts. The junior Navy Corpsman deployed with me asked for a consult on a patient who had been experiencing knee pain for 3 days, unrelieved by non-steroidal, anti-inflammatory medications (NSAIDS). Upon examination, I noted that the calf of the affected leg was larger than that of the non-affected leg. After a thorough exam and comprehensive history, I consulted my physician preceptor with concerns of a deep vein thrombosis (DVT) and requested authorization for an ultrasound, which was approved and subsequently revealed a very large clot in the popliteal vein. Even though the likelihood of a DVT was slim, my instinct, training, and experience resulted in prompt treatment and averted a potentially life-threatening complication.

During my 20-year military career, I was deployed numerous times, from the first Gulf War to Operation Iraqi Freedom. I was always proud of my service because I knew I made a difference and without me some of those men and women might not have come home. I chose to retire after 20 years and 7 months of service when the realization that my next promotion, which was inevitable, would mean I was no longer going to be involved in patient care, and I would be relegated to a strictly administrative function.

My military experience has provided me with the maturity and life experiences that will allow me to adapt well to the rigorous scholastic environment of the Physician Assistant program. In the beginning, I hit a few bumps grade wise because the shift from "real life" to the academic world proved to be a challenging transition. After joining several study groups, my study skills and confidence improved dramatically over the next few months. My extensive experience in a clinical setting will also be a huge benefit during clinical rotations. A lesson learned early in my career was that in order to be a good leader, you must first be a good follower. I earned numerous awards and decorations during my time in the Air Force, including two Meritorious Service Awards, a Humanitarian Service Award, and several Airman, Noncommissioned Officer, and Senior Noncommissioned Officer of the Quarter Awards.

Although any career in healthcare is rewarding, I hope to fulfill my lifelong goal of becoming a PA and reaching the lofty heights achieved by my inspiration Jim. Upon graduation from PA school, it is my intention to apply for a job with either the Veterans Administration or with a military facility as a contracted provider. I know I have more to give back to the military and feel the best way to do that is to continue to provide the best healthcare possible to the men and women of the Armed Services and our Veterans.

Essay 10 (825 words)

"Ready! Droppin' in 3 . . . 2 . . . 1," I called to the videographers and photographers below me. The whiteout conditions on that January day had hindered our filming efforts and, as the weather broke, I knew that my chances to complete the maneuver were limited. My heart raced as I looked toward the edge of the cliff, but I pushed doubt and fear from my mind and focused on making a perfect landing. With my snowboard pointing downhill, I visualized my landing and followed through with precision and confidence.

Throughout my ten-year career as a professional snowboarder, jumping off cliffs had become routine, and I believed in myself and in my abilities. Aware that hesitation results in accidents, I continually pushed myself to advance and excel. Understanding my mind and body was vital to my success, and I became obsessed with health, wellness, and healing. Now, as I prepare to become a physician assistant, I approach a different cliff in my life, but the same principles of preparation, practice, commitment, and confidence still apply.

After identifying my goal of becoming a PA, I availed myself of opportunities to explore the healthcare field and advance my education. One of my most rewarding experiences was volunteering at the People's Health Clinic in Park City, Utah, where uninsured individuals receive free care. My responsibilities included taking patients' vitals and escorting them to exam rooms, and I experienced great satisfaction when patients expressed their gratitude for the clinic and for my services. Volunteering at this clinic solidified my desire to provide healthcare services and use my talents and skills to give back to my community.

I have always had a strong desire to make a difference in the world, and I found a way to achieve this personal goal seven years ago. After touring a homeless shelter called The Road Home, I discovered that the residents' most requested item was new socks, so I established the non-profit organization, Stoked On Socks. We collect new pairs of socks and donate them to those in need, proving again that one person can make a difference in the lives of others. When I complete my PA training and join this profession, I will continue to make a difference.

In my current position as a respiratory assistant, I enjoy working with patients. I once fitted a woman with a CPAP mask and educated her about obstructive sleep apnea and the use of the CPAP machine. She described her sleep problems and the negative impact on her life, and I reassured her that the doctor had ordered this course of treatment because he believed the therapy would help her. A few days later, she excitedly reported that she was sleeping better and no longer needed naps during the day. This was one of many experiences where I would have preferred becoming more involved in the patient's continued treatment. My current position as a respiratory assistant allows me significant autonomy while working with patients, and should I need additional guidance, a respiratory therapist is always just a phone call away. As a PA, I will work in an autonomous environment where I will fulfill my desire to diagnose, treat, and provide follow-up care.

Providing healthcare services in times of distress is a valuable contribution. As a youth group volunteer, I helped provide services when another adult leader fell and split his chin. We were hours away from the nearest hospital, but we were fortunate to have a doctor with us who had brought his suture kit. The doctor cleaned the wound and sutured the man's chin. He asked if I would like to put a few sutures in, and with the patient's permission, I proceeded. Although I appreciated being involved, I wanted to be the one doing all of the sutures, treating the wound, and removing the sutures after healing had taken place. As a PA, I will have the skills and knowledge necessary to respond to emergencies and remain involved throughout the treatment and follow-up process.

With every step of my preparation to serve as a PA, my passion and desire increases. I have shadowed numerous physician assistants and enjoyed watching their interactions with patients. While shadowing a PA in neurology, I watched as she and the doctor reviewed a patient's brain scan and pointed out small irregularities. In a recent anatomy course, I had thoroughly studied the identical portions of the brain and the areas of the body that are affected by them. I instantly applied this classroom knowledge to the real world of healthcare, and it was exhilarating to make that connection.

I know that my career as a PA will be exciting and fulfilling. Attending a physician assistant program will be extremely intense, but the principles I used to achieve the skill level of a professional snowboarder will also apply to this aspect of my life. I will be determined, dedicated, and committed to my goal of becoming the best PA I can possibly be.

Essay 11 (893 words)

I was born in a small industrial city in Russia. My father was a cardiovascular surgeon and my mother is a Feldsher (equivalent of Physician Assistant (PA) in the US). My father left our family when I was 2 years old, and I never met him again. But I was always told that he is a hero, because he saves people's lives. I remember my mom working hard on two jobs to give me the best education she could. Thus, I was a busy kid, and at the age of 9 I had graduated from musical school in class piano, took English lessons in one of the private schools, dance classes, and all the while still attending my elementary school. Since my mother was busy all the time, I was taken care of mostly by my grandmother who lived with us. We were very close to each other. Then, when I was a teenager, she suffered a stroke. She survived, but after that was sick for a year. It was a painful time for both my mother and myself. I was 15, and now it was I who helped take care of my nana every day after I got back from school. I saw her in pain, not being able to eat, or use the bathroom without help. That year of grief absolutely opened my eyes on what I wanted to do with my life—I wanted to help people.

During my final year of high school, I volunteered at the Skin and Venereal Diseases Hospital where my mother worked. I remember seeing her with the patients and how she would ask them to smile. Later she explained it as a trick, "If you ask them to smile then they feel much better after doing that than after taking the medicine." I observed and helped doctors and nurses perform procedures on patients. I learned medical terminology, how to collect lab specimens, and obtain vital signs. I walked patients to the tests, helped them with dressing up, taking baths, and skin care. But the most valuable thing that I learned is to keep your heart open with patients who suffer from pain and disease. They need to be not only treated with procedures and pills, but also to be heard and emotionally supported.

At 17 years old, I moved to the bigger city and the capital of the country—Moscow. It was a time of new opportunities and choosing my career direction. My oldest cousin who lived there and worked in television had influenced me to become a journalist. I studied journalism at Moscow State Humanitarian University for 5 years. This opportunity gave me invaluable experience with the skills of gathering, analyzing, and delivering information and putting it into a format that is understood by others. I learned how to verify facts, to be trustworthy with sensitive information, to be able to relate well to a wide variety of people, and to adapt to constantly changing circumstances. But soon I started to realize this was not what I dreamed about doing with my life. By working as a journalist I was serving people with information, but I wanted not just to serve them, but to help them—big difference! I decided to take a break in my life and find my true path.

At 22, I participated in the International Student Exchange Program. I came to the United States and decided to start all over again. I always knew that I wanted to work with people, to make them feel better. Therefore, I pursued a Bachelors Degree in Biomolecular Sciences—the first stepping-stone in my medical career. During my first year of study I had to become proficient in English very quickly, thus my grades suffered in the beginning. Yet, after a lot of hard work, my English improved and studying became easier. Soon, I became a Dean's List student and was awarded scholarships for academic achievement.

During this time, I was able to shadow a PA in the Emergency Department. I was impressed by his work with critically ill patients and resolving acute emergencies. I have seen and followed patients from their admission through discharge from the hospital.

My other shadowing experience was with an Orthopedic PA from Connecticut Children's Medical Center. I observed him working with patients during regular office exams and also in the Operating Room where he and the rest of the surgery team performed limb lengthening and deformity correction.

Presently, I work as an Emergency Medical Technician in the Emergency Department. This experience is teaching me how to work under extreme conditions of stress. I am also always interested to learn from observing the PAs and MDs who work there, asking them to explain x-rays and CT scan images. I want to become a PA because of a long path that started with my mom and the example she gave me. Like her, I want to enjoy the direct contact with patients and most of all to be able to help people who are in serious need. I am 26 now, married, and a stepmother myself to three beautiful girls. I am ready to spend my life dedicated to helping other families like mine and to achieving a life/work balance. I know that the best way to accomplish both of these goals is to become a PA.

Essay 12 (864 words)

"Rand missus?" The boy held out his tiny grimy hands, eagerly, hopefully. Most striking was the smaller child standing next to him, a gaping hole extending up from his split upper lip. I handed the boy the change I had, knowing it could do little to improve their situation, but wanting to do something. Their hopeful, expectant faces created a poignant image that remains with me, even now, 15 years later. It was during this trip to the war ravaged capital of Mozambique, as a young exchange student studying in South Africa, that I first became truly mindful of the physical consequences of poverty. I felt quite helpless at that time and wished I could do more for them. My brief encounter with them, and similar experiences while in South Africa, made me realize that I didn't want to be helpless. I wanted to make an impact in the lives of those around me. Specifically, I decided that I wanted to pursue a career path, where I could contribute to the health and well-being of my community.

Returning from my studies abroad, I changed my major to Anthropology. I knew that I wanted to go into some sort of health field, and felt strongly that understanding people and the cultural context in which they exist would be a good start. I also completed all of the pre-requisites for applying to medical school. Following graduation, rather than medical school, I chose to obtain a graduate degree in public health at the University of Utah. This proved to be a natural complement to my studies in anthropology and a very rewarding experience. I really felt like I had found my niche and hoped it would provide me the opportunity to make a positive contribution to the community.

I was fortunate to get a job with the Utah Department of Health, Office of Epidemiology, in the sexually transmitted disease (STD) surveillance program. My responsibilities included working collaboratively with a variety of health care professionals, including medical providers, public health nurses and social workers to ensure that all those testing positive for reportable STDs were properly treated and partner follow-up was conducted. My co-worker and I met with and interviewed minors with STDs in detention facilities and drug treatment centers across the Wasatch Front. We also developed an educational presentation on STDs and their prevention which we presented at various facilities across the state. Seeing the frequency of STDs in specific youth populations, I wrote and was awarded a CDC grant to assess the magnitude of the problem in Utah. Through this grant, we were able to actively screen for STDs and pregnancy in over a thousand at-risk youth in detention facilities, drug treatment centers, and a homeless youth clinic. We also wrote and administered a survey to those we tested, in order to better understand the types of high risk behaviors that were increasing the risk of infection in this population. This also provided an opportunity to meet with and discuss individually, strategies to help these teens stay safe and healthy in the future. At times, our interactions were emotional and challenging, but I always felt that we were able to make a positive difference in the lives of these youth.

My career as an epidemiologist was cut short due to personal health problems. In retrospect I believe these health issues were a mixed blessing for two reasons. First, I had the opportunity to be a patient, a role that I'll admit to not relishing. I experienced the relief and gratitude a patient feels when treated with dignity, sincere concern and respect. I also was the recipient of care that was lacking in these qualities. These experiences had a profound impact on my view of the responsibility health care providers have to their patients. I understand that healing a patient physically is not always possible. However, I do believe that the best care is always delivered compassionately, respectfully and takes into consideration the individual's entire health picture. Secondly, the time away from my work as an epidemiologist allowed for significant introspection as to whether I felt I was accomplishing my personal and professional goals. From this I realized that what I really wanted was to work more closely with patients than what I was able to as an epidemiologist.

As my health improved and I began to assess the options available to me, I quickly came to the conclusion that becoming a physician assistant would allow me to fulfill my goals. I believe that my life thus far has really prepared me for this profession. The role the physician assistant plays in health care delivery is perfectly suited to both the innate and acquired skills I possess. I believe that both my anthropological and public health training along with the maturity and commitment I possess as a non-traditional student will help me succeed as a PA student and physician assistant. I know that once I become a physician assistant, my curiosity, ability to actively listen and engage, along with empathy and my sincere desire to serve others will enable me to make a significant and positive impact on the health and well-being of my patients.

Essay 13 (520 words)

The Physician Assistant (PA) profession fulfills a unique niche in medicine. The aspects of this career that makes it so interesting and fitting for me are: the team dynamics of working with physicians, nurses, and other health care professionals, the opportunity and flexibility to work in different subspecialty areas, and the ability to spend more time with patients than the supervising physician. I particularly am drawn to the dynamic of collaborating with physicians to ensure quality care is given. The particular aspect of the PA profession

I desire is the ability to be trained as a generalist and further the education to a specialty if I desire.

Commitment, resilience, and the skill sets I have developed can only be discussed by referencing my prior experiences. Accepting Teach For America's offer to teach in low-income schools across the country, where I did not know anyone, was pivotal. My level of commitment was tested and approved. I became devoted to helping an underserved population, even though it meant leaving my friends, family, and everything I've known behind. The resilience of teaching came in the ninety-hour work weeks, driving students home, and relentless pursuit of success of my students. The best part of the Teach For America opportunity was being challenged with tough circumstances and few resources yet preserving through them to get results. This program and my previous experiences have proven that I am committed to my passions and resilient to persevere through obstacles. Through my experiences I have exemplified my strong interpersonal skills, self-determination, organization, time management, and empathy towards others. My ability to effectively and concisely communicate with the individuals was a vital component to success. Simultaneously, my organization and time management led to my student and athlete's success, which was fueled by my empathy, passion and determination to relentlessly ensure they were reaching their goals.

One thing I am improving upon is my multitasking. In college and high school, I did an impeccable job juggling work, school, athletics, and multiple volunteer activities. However, I never could fully devote to an activity that I felt strongly. Through teaching, I've worked to not stretch myself, which led to great successes with my students. My involvement working with diverse communities has been a lifelong commitment through teaching, Special Olympics, caring for patients in home care, and assisting women in a battered shelter. I excel in places where I am stretched to creatively and professionally care for individuals different from myself. I am committed to continuing to do so in the PA profession.

Pacific's PA program offers unique and exceptional opportunities to hone my skills in the medical field and provide exceptional healthcare to diverse populations. The opportunities to improve my Spanish and provide international healthcare while in school are two of the ways Pacific will support me in working with diverse populations in the medical profession. Pacific's impeccable reputation to successfully prepare students for success on the boards and beyond is essential for my goal attainment. Thus, this program would help me to not only successfully develop my skills to be a PA but also to thrive into the future within the profession.

Essay 14 (883 words)

Some of us are fortunate enough to have a person enter our life that has such a profound impact that it forever changes the direction of our lives. For me this was my brother-in-law's mother. She had an amazing capacity for giving that was evident from the first time I met her. Judy was a nurse who spent her life dedicated to helping others, ultimately becoming one of the first hospice nurses in northeastern Ohio, working with the Hospice of the Western Reserve. I did not realize the magnitude of her impact on my life until last year when she lost her battle with brain cancer. I was moved to tears as person after person stood up at her funeral and spoke of the positive impact she had on their lives and the comfort she provided. It was at this moment that my life changed forever.

I had known for some time I had to make a change. My entire career had been spent working in the corporate world where all that matters is the bottom line. I needed to find a way to help others and, more importantly, to make a difference. In the months following Judy's funeral, I struggled to find the correct fit. Soon after I had my first experience with a physician assistant and everything became clear. After suffering a stress fracture in my leg I was referred to an orthopedist. The PA that did my initial assessment was truly amazing. She spent a great deal of time explaining my injury and discussing my x-ray and MRI, covering all the structures involved. I immediately began investigating the PA profession and became more excited the more I learned. The teamwork, the collaboration, and the autonomy all caught my attention. These were all aspects of working that I not only enjoyed, but also excelled at during my 20 years working in information technology. After months of considering a career change I knew I wanted to become a PA.

Once I made the decision to pursue a new career as a PA I pursued as much knowledge and exposure as I could. I immediately contacted the Ohio Association of Physician Assistants to obtain a list of PAs to shadow. I was fortunate to be put in contact with a great PA working in Orthopedics. Shadowing Sarah allowed me to see first-hand the positive impact PAs have on their patients. I spent a good deal of time with her and really got to know her patients. I found myself taking an interest in Sarah's patients' care and looked forward to seeing them again and following their progress. The PA shadowing was such a positive experience I wanted to do more. Unfortunately with 20 years of IT experience I found it difficult to find a patient-centered position. I decided to volunteer at a local hospital in the trauma unit. The volunteer position has allowed me to interact with patients and gain insight into the hospital environment. Just seeing the joy brought to a patient by the simple act of getting a warm blanket or a glass of water has provided me with a sense of purpose.

The biggest obstacle in my path is my early academic performance. Despite taking the college prep curriculum in high school, I was not challenged academically. I graduated near the top of my class with minimal amount of work. Once I started college it became apparent this approach would not be successful. I lacked the necessary study skills but was too proud to reach out for help. Prior to my second year, my parents divorced and I was forced to move out on my own. It seemed that overnight my focus shifted from being simply a student to needing to support myself and pay rent. I struggled to balance school with working enough to meet my basic expenses. My school attendance and grades both suffered. The low point came when I was dismissed from Ohio State University. This was the wakeup I desperately needed. I used this time to reflect and focus on getting my life together. I began a job at a computer store, then worked my way into the corporate IT world where I was promoted several times and moved into positions with increasing responsibility. When I returned to school I was more mature and ready to succeed. I had learned to manage my time, set priorities, and most importantly to ask for help when I need it. My grades over the past several years reflect this maturity and focus. I have rededicated myself since returning to complete my PA prerequisites, making the necessary sacrifices to maintain a 4.0 GPA, all while still working full time.

While I may have a nontraditional background, my experiences and adversities have prepared me well for this next, challenging stage in my life. I have the high level of commitment and dedication necessary to be successful. Most importantly I have the desire and passion to not just help others but to make a difference in their lives. I have been asked numerous times if it is hard to give up the lucrative career I built in IT to return to school. The answer is always a simple "no," because I now realize this is what I am meant to do.

Essay 15 (860 words)

At 17 my doctor diagnosed me with Scheuermann's kyphoscoliosis and a spinal curvature of 90 degrees. I underwent a full thoracic-lumbar spinal fusion from vertebrae C3 to L4 at Shriners Hospital. From the moment I was extubated in the operating room and through the week of re-learning to walk, the nurses, surgeons, and medical staff gave me comfort and hope in a time of unbearable pain. When initially looking at the X-Rays with new hardware screwed into my spine, I was instantly intrigued how one procedure could change my posture and my life. Through the course of my recovery, I dreamed of the possibility I too could change lives through medicine. Many experiences influenced my desire to choose the Physician Assistant (PA) profession as my means of helping people through healthcare.

Although I was unprepared to excel at such a competitive level when I began college, my knowledge flourished after gaining healthcare experience at a level one trauma hospital. After my sophomore year, I shadowed Medical Doctors (MD) and inadvertently the PAs at Tampa General Hospital (TGH) to explore and learn about medical professions. I was unaware of the PAs' role but impressed I could not distinguish between the knowledge and technique of the MDs and PAs. While rounding with the critical care team, I noticed the PAs had more time to assess and connect with their patients. One of the PAs was so personable to her patients that many times patients preferred to see her instead of their doctor. The PAs taught me various treatments and pathologies they manage day to day such as tracheostomies and sepsis. They also exemplified their responsibilities when responding to a code blue and managing the airway of a patient. I now understand the important role of the members of the PA-MD team model and know that the more personal patient interaction of the PA is the perfect profession for me.

After deciding to become a PA, I aspired to expose myself to many fields in the medical arena to prepare for the diversity of the profession. I began this journey by working in clinical research with the anesthesiology and surgery departments at TGH and was intuitively involved in the academic side of medicine. Our team collaborated with the University of South Florida College of Medicine and focused on innovative surgical techniques, novel burn dressings, and varied analgesic regimens; leading to numerous publications. My patient interaction with research linked patient care to the constantly changing world of medicine. In an effort to provide the most recent and effective care to patients, being involved in clinical research is important to me as a future PA.

I continued my mission by volunteering as an emergency medical responder at Florida State University. I learned and demonstrated the urgency and alertness one must possess when arriving at an emergency. My skills were put to the test when I arrived at the scene of an unconscious male who fell off his skateboard resulting in a large laceration to his head. Arriving and assessing the scene to distinguish between a medical or trauma emergency and acting accordingly made these types of calls suspenseful and challenging. This experience will help me with decision making as a PA when handling stressful cases and making critical diagnoses.

My view of medicine expanded beyond my comfortable borders after traveling to the mountains of Buff Bay Jamaica with a diverse team of medical professionals. In a span of ten days we diagnosed and treated over 700 Jamaicans who otherwise had no access to healthcare. Prior to going on this trip the need in underprivileged countries carried no relevance in my life. This trip opened my eyes to the reality that people all over the world live where little to no health education or resources exists everyday. The overwhelming gratuity and constant joy of the Jamaican people, despite limited material possessions made every day at clinic inspirational. I returned to America realizing that my motivation to become a PA was not one of self-gain but of service to those in need.

Finally, I expanded my role at TGH by working as a patient care technician on the neuro-surgery floor. This job led me to care for diverse patients ranging from stroke to psychiatric patients and the unique opportunity to care for patients recovering from spinal fusion surgery. My firsthand experience was invaluable for connecting with patients who were often doubtful or anxious about their recovery from spine surgery... This opportunity gave a sense of comfort and hope to my patients that believed no one else understood what they were going through; a quality I hope to display as a PA.

My preparation for becoming a PA has allowed me to view medicine through multiple lenses. I have seen that despite the diverse environments where healthcare occurs, the mission remains the same: providing a tangible way to love and heal the hurting. My long term goals as a PA are twofold: working in surgery and actively participating in local and international medical missions. If given the opportunity, I am confident my clinical experience has afforded me maturity, drive, and focus to excel in PA school.

Essay 16 (769 words)

The journey began at a mere four years old. The dream and goal were set by eight. The sacrifice, focus, and dedication that would be necessary were realized by ten. Great success came by sixteen and a bittersweet feeling by 23.

"Lub-dub, lub-dub, lub-dub"; I could feel my heart beat. I could faintly hear "U-S-A, U-S-A, go Danielle!" echoing from the bleachers as time counted down in the championship fight. "Three, two, one, ding"; I had become the Pan American Champion at 16 years old. These are the sounds and feelings that have filled my soul since 8 years old and have stayed the same; training after training, kick after kick, year after year, through the past fifteen years of taekwondo competitions. All the missed football games, dances, and sleep, combined with long drives and extra training, paid off. Eventually, they led me to a training partnership at the 2008 Beijing Olympics, a spot on two national teams, and 5th place at the 2009 World Championships in Taekwondo. More importantly, I walked away with skills and intangible life experiences which, paired with my parent's unparalleled love, have made me into the person I am today and have given me a clear vision for the future.

Discovering the greatness of having a team, the joys of travel abroad, and the importance of taking care of your body, are three of the greatest gifts that taekwondo has given me. Despite taekwondo being an individual sport, our team is the backbone of our individual success. We feed off each other's energy, athletic knowledge, and motivation. We all have different upbringings, values, and personalities, but love and support each other like a second family.

In addition to my friends and teammates locally, travel to over 15 countries has introduced me to different cultures and great people around the globe. Eating local foods and experiencing local traditions have made me appreciate every way of life. Thanks to my travels, I have made good friends in Guatemala, Denmark, and Mexico.

All of my travels have been meaningful. However, my most impactful trip was to Brazil. I remember driving from the airport to the hotel. We passed mountainsides of adobe-like one-bedroom homes with dirt floors, no running water, and children running barefoot through the streets. For the first time in my life, I felt powerless, sadness, and a rejuvenated desire to help.

As an athlete, understanding your body and training it to achieve maximum efficiency is key for longevity. It is incredible how our bodies can withstand strenuous exercise and how each body system functions together to maintain optimal performance. Throughout my years as an athlete, cutting weight and pushing myself to the max has taught me the best ways to fuel, strengthen, heal, and rest my body. All of these experiences have helped me to better understand myself and the type of work I would enjoy. But, the daunting question still remained; what did I want to be when I "grew up"?

I knew I enjoyed my science classes. I knew that the intricate physiology of the human body amazed me and that I found fulfillment in helping people from all backgrounds. However, it was not until mid-junior year, when a fellow classmate and I were conversing about our future career goals, that I first heard of a Physician Assistant. He proceeded to explain to me what a PA did and the path to become one. Suddenly, a feeling of relief came over me; "Wow that sounds perfect!"

In the following months I shadowed several Physician Assistants. A PA at Miami Children's Hospital became my mentor. Not only did she let me shadow her, but I got to accompany her to hospital meetings. She encouraged me to start working with patients. Now, after 9 months as an orthopedic tech assistant, my passion to help people has only grown.

Although I lack extensive direct patient experience, if given the opportunity, I will work diligently to become an important member of the healthcare team. I am prepared for a rigorous course of study and excited for all the practical applications. As a future Physician Assistant, I look forward to working both independently and collaboratively with supervising physicians in a challenging environment. I want to provide a better quality of life for my patients.

As my dad, a speech and language pathologist in nursing homes, once told me, "No matter how long you have been working, never forget to treat every patient and person with purpose and compassion." These are the words I live by as I embark on my new journey to becoming a successful Physician Assistant.

Essay 17 (803 words)

Jambo! Welcome to Kenya—my native land. Strolling through the vast streets of Africa, a few right and left turns takes you to the baseball fields of Kisumu Elementary School. It is the perfect day, with the sunshine giving enough warmth as to rid the wind chill, for the title game against the rival elementary school. Thus far, at the end of the 3rd quarter, both schools are tied and I am the last player up to bat. With fierce determination and a bat in my hands, I studied the thrower with a glance that spoke louder than words. Two fast pitches and he had knocked me off my base. Yet even when the pitcher held the ball in his hand with the confidence to settle my team's fate, I resolutely maintained my conviction of winning the game. I swung the bat vigorously as the ball came to me and…and the ball flew to the sky. We won; my team had won!

Contemplating back to that memory I am reminded of just how immensely different the achievements of a child versus those of an adult are. As a child, I was overwhelmed by a mere baseball game win. However, today my ambitions are to prepare myself for a new, more challenging goal; to become a physician assistant. At the tender age of 8, I arrived to the United States along with my family to pursue the "American Dream". Only those who are immigrants can comprehend the adversities of adjusting to a new language, a new atmosphere and a whole new lifestyle. The first day of 5th grade was the longest day of my life. I still remember how I didn't go to the bathroom for the entire day because none of the kids understood me when I asked where the "loo" was. Although, I eventually learned to grow into this new lifestyle and, while I will never forget my background, I learned to adapt to my new environment. Thankfully, along with the hardships, came rewards. Being in the "land of opportunity," meant that now I had the opportunity to strive towards any goal I could possibly conceive of.

As I went on to high school and college, my desire to be a PA has been continually reinforced. I was able to gain firsthand experience in patient care quite early in my college years. One of the most satisfying volunteer experiences I had was when I was an emergency medical technician at Montclair University's EMS for over a year. In that time, I learned that medicine is nothing like I had thought in the past. I still remember, only a few months into my training, I saw my first critical patient. "Lub dub, lub dub, lub dub". The man had Ischemic heart disease. I found that he died just minutes' after he was discharged to the ER. He just laid there—pale, empty, lifeless—just laid there. Although this transpired at least twenty times on episodes of House M.D., actually seeing first-hand this situation was a really life changing experience for me.

Forthwith, the satisfaction of being an EMT diminished considerably. I realized that I tended to patients for particular ailments but then I was to never see them. I would begin to wonder; what happened to them; will the ketoac-idotic patient that I took care of last year live to see today? Perhaps I would never know, though I sincerely wish I did. As a physician assistant, I would be able to provide comprehensive care to my patients and be available to them for on-going consultation, which is one of the essential reasons why I aspire to become a PA.

One of the most interesting experiences I encountered during my under-graduate college was taking part in research. Though I certainly enjoyed classroom learning and all it had to offer, I excelled when it came to hands-on learning. Research with Dr. Adams on inhibition of SinV Virus, responsible for the Sindbis fever, prevalent in Kenya and other parts of Africa, was truly intriguing so much that I devoted more time into research then I had ever thought possible. The one aspect of medical research that still amazes me is knowing that I, a mere college biology student, understands something that no one has grasped yet. Research is what I can take pride in, though monotonous and tedious, I feel as if I am accomplishing something great, even if it may be miniscule in the grand scheme of things.

Being a physician assistant would give me the opportunity to fuse all my interests and career goals together. While research is invaluable to the path of dis-covery, volunteering as an EMT has shown me that patient care is where I really belong since I would be able to fulfill my long-term career goal best that way.

Essay 18 (339 words)

Several years ago, I had the opportunity to reevaluate my life plans. I realized I wanted to begin a career in the medical field, and entered a medical assisting program. During the training, I learned of various medical careers, and became captivated with the physician assistant profession. I discovered it is one of the few medical professions that not only allows involvement in patient care, but also in diagnosis and treatment.

At present, I work in a family practice office as a back office medical assistant and scribe. This means that I also have the opportunity to work alongside the doctor during each office visit. I add history, diagnoses, physical exam details and treatment plans to the office visit note while the doctor is performing the exam. Meanwhile, I also scan the electronic medical record for information that would be important to that particular visit. For example, when the doctor is considering certain medications that may affect kidney function, I look to ensure the patient has no diminished kidney function on recent lab results. I question the patient and doctor for clarification, and I propose diagnostic tests or treatments for the doctor's consideration. Observing the doctor's ability to determine when a firm hand or compassionate hand is needed has also been extremely enlightening.

I have also had the occasion to see the healthcare field from a patient's perspective. A recent diagnosis of simultaneous ovarian cancer and endometrial cancer has allowed me to see the difference a compassionate caregiver can make to a patient who is in the midst of a serious diagnosis. It has also taught me the value of early diagnosis and treatment.

I currently live in a medically underserved rural area, and understand many of the challenges of such an area. In particular, I am reminded of one elderly diabetic patient who could not afford to drive the few miles to pick up his insulin at the office where I worked. I brought it to his tiny house on my way home. That day, he also asked me for information on diabetic diets; I brought a book to him the next day.

I would prefer to work in family practice as a physician assistant where I could care for patients with varied conditions and backgrounds. I look forward to future challenges and rewards of a lifelong career as a physician assistant.

Essay 19 (1346 words)

"A PA helped save my daughter's life" exclaimed my co-worker Christy. She detailed how the persistence and advocacy of a PA at the ER had been instrumental in diagnosing her daughter with Kawasaki syndrome. As she spoke, I was struck—yet again—by the dedication of this PA; not unlike that of the many other PAs I had contacted in prior months. Though I had been exploring the profession for some time already, it was this defining moment that truly cemented my desire to become a PA.

Growing up outside Bombay, India, my late grandfather had been our town's first doctor; I grew up hearing stories of his love for people and medicine. My grandmother— who suffered a stroke and diabetes—let me to "help" her take insulin shots and medication. Though I was young, these experiences left a strong impression; it was during this time my love of service and healthcare was born.

Growing up in India was a wonderful experience; I learned to interact and live with people of diverse perspectives, cultures, languages and religions. In

March 1993, due to ongoing religious rifts, a string of bombs were set off in downtown Bombay. My father's office building was a target; he was trapped for hours before being rescued. Though he suffered only minor injuries, my family was shaken to its core; we immigrated to Canada shortly thereafter.

In Canada, my father was unable to find a job and succumbed to depression and alcoholism. I started working at 15, to help support my mother and younger brother. Though far from ideal, this situation instilled in me excellent time management skills, and a determination to excel. I learned to balance paid work with strong academics and community service. This included volunteer positions at an animal shelter, a sexual and domestic violence hotline, a local hospital, an opera house, and with local environmental groups. Working at the crisis hotline and at the hospital, I realized my true desire was to serve people through healthcare—though I was still unsure of the route I would take.

When accepted to the University of Toronto, I made the difficult decision to continue living at home and supporting my family. Since my decision made me ineligible to receive financial aid, I took on a second job to fund my education. This was a crippling period in my life: emotionally, physically, financially and academically. Despite a strong desire to excel, and an inherent love of learning, I simply did not have the time or the means to demonstrate my academic ability. Coping with my father's disease—and his increasing verbal and physical outbursts—eroded our family finances and all sense of stability. A heavy work schedule, combined with the increased financial burden of education and a competitive academic environment, meant I could not perform at a level that reflected my true academic abilities. Though dropping out of school would have alleviated much stress, I persisted, determined to graduate in good standing, in my chosen field. Though it was the most challenging time of my life, it taught me maturity, adaptability, and most of all, perseverance. I graduated in good standing in 2006, and moved to Texas shortly after.

In 2007 I began work at Cogenics, as part of team that provided molecular biology services to a wide range of clients. The technical and logistical challenges of the job were enjoyable; as was the opportunity to expand on knowledge acquired in university. In 2009, I moved to Biotics Research Corporation (BRC), a respected nutraceutical company that manufactured over a 100 unique dietary supplements. Working at BRC was a tremendous growing experience. As the only Quality Assurance (QA) Coordinator, I supervised a team of 8 QA Associates, as well as acted as a liaison between the Board of Directors and company-wide QA activity. In this fast-paced environment, I learnt crisis management, how to identify and solve unique problems, and most of all, how to effectively work in high stress situations while maintaining my composure and the integrity of my role. The health-related aspects of this job strongly rekindled my desire to work in healthcare; I knew without doubt, that a future profession based on a medical model of education was my goal.

Shortly after I began work at BRC in 2009, my husband was treated for an eye injury by a PA at our local ER. I was impressed with her depth of knowledge, calm demeanor and the ease with which she worked alongside the doctor to treat my husband. She was happy to tell me about her journey into the PA profession; that very night began my quest into understanding the profession more fully. I joined the AAPA, and contacted as many PAs as possible. In the many phone and e-mail conversations that ensued, two similarities stood out—all loved their chosen profession and the team oriented nature of their jobs—both were traits I strongly valued in any future profession. In shadowing five PAs, I was amazed at the range and complexity of specialties they practice in—from the ICU to cardiovascular surgery—and also at the unique relationship that exist between each PA and supervising physician. It was also during this time I met Christy, and experienced the defining moment that led to this application.

I quit my job in June 2010, and returned to school full-time; I wanted to prove my academic capability and become a more competitive PA candidate. Since then I have completed 42 hours in PA pre-requisites with a 4.0 GPA. I also volunteer in the community: as an adult "English as a Second Language" (ESL) teacher; at Houston Hospice; and most recently at Omega House.

As an adult ESL teacher in an underserved community, I develop curriculum and teach adults to speak and write English. All of my students are immigrants, who—as I once did—cope with various levels of cultural isolation. Being able to empathize with their situation has helped me not only be a teacher, but a life-coach and cheerleader of sorts. I am proud to say that with my help, many have dramatically improved their language skills; some have even gone on to find jobs or complete their GEDs—goals they never thought possible.

At Houston Hospice, I have the honor and privilege of interacting with patients in the final chapter of their lives. Learning to deal with death in medicine was a challenge. Here, I learnt that being a good care-giver means more than administering treatments— it means offering empathy and comfort as well. It saddens me that PAs are still unable to practice in this area of medicine; if given the opportunity, I hope to one day be part of the growing PA movement that is trying this.

While at Houston Hospice, a lead nurse recommended I volunteer at Omega House, where she had previously been Director of Nursing. Omega House is a residential hospice for people in the late stages of HIV/AIDS; volunteers contribute almost 70% of patient care. Here, I have had the opportunity to serve with patients in many ways: by socializing and interacting with them; cooking meals, changing clothes and diapers; helping feed, bathe and attend to personal hygiene; as well helping nurses chart daily progress, remove catheters and administer medication. Both hospice positions have given me a deep sense of fulfillment, and deepened my longing to be able to serve and treat patients in a greater capacity.

I want to be a PA because I want to be part of a growing profession that is hands-on, practical, challenging and constantly evolving. Working with supervising physicians means exciting opportunities to acquire new skills and knowledge and the ability to practice in more than one area of healthcare. With my strong love of learning, a genuine desire to serve patients and the skills acquired through my life experiences, I feel that I am a strong candidate for the PA profession. If given the opportunity, I also hope to contribute to the PA community by being an advocate for the profession, and by helping educate future generations of PAs.

Essay 20 (856 words)

Some events alter the course of your life and drive you towards a clear goal. At the age of eleven, my friends and I were playing soccer when my friend fell and split his forehead on a rock. In a fraction of a second, blood drenched his whole face and I leapt into action, tending to my friend who was in a state of panic. Despite my own rattled nerves, I pulled out my handkerchief and applied pressure to his wound—a response that was second nature after having observed my mother, a nurse, do the same thing dozens of times. I instructed my friends to call the nurse while I assured him that he would be fine. I felt his nerves begin to calm, and by the time the nurses arrived, my uniform was soaked in blood. They continued to apply pressure to keep him from bleeding to death before he safely reached the ER. From that day forward, my clear and driving passion was medicine. I witnessed firsthand how practicing medicine was not only about prescribing medication or performing surgery but also about caring for people and applying information that could ultimately save lives.

My passion for medicine was deepened when a car accident hospitalized my mother my freshman year of college. During that time, I ended up paying more attention to my recovering mother and my struggling family, working full-time at Whole Foods Market to support my family. My grades suffered, serving as the wakeup call that made me realize that failing to perform my best helped no one and led me to develop better self-management under adverse circumstances. I learned to prioritize my coursework and proudly graduated with a 3.26 grade point average.

Two years ago, tragedy reared its ugly head again when my mother was diagnosed with saddle pulmonary embolism and was admitted at Beth Israel Hospital for two weeks. Our family was grief-stricken at the thought of losing our mother, yet nearly every visit we found her chatting good-naturedly with her PA. They developed a friendship, and I saw what a difference the PA made not only in caring for my mother's physical health but for her mental health as well. The way she accompanied my mother's every step until her recovery triggered my decision to pursue a career as a physician assistant.

My desire to become a PA was enhanced by my research during my senior year of college with a fellow classmate under the guidance of Dr. Mande Holford. Our research focused on Solid Phase Peptide Synthesis of Teretoxins snails and their characterization through HPLC and mass spectrometry. Even more than our findings, we gained valuable lessons on teamwork, diligence, and patience despite setbacks along the way. I was fascinated by the potential of snail toxins to alleviate chronic pain in HIV and cancer patients, and my interest in HIV patients caused me to search for ways to contribute to their well-being. I found the perfect opportunity to join two medical trips in regions severely affected by the HIV epidemic: the African nation of Tanzania and La Ceiba, Honduras. From my first trip, I worked in a rehabilitation center for HIV/ AIDS orphans where I met a teary eyed three-year-old boy named Winner, a HIV infected orphan. From the time I first picked him up, it was clear to me that, more than medicine, this boy was desperately in need of love and affection. The highlight of every day was seeing Winner run to me with his arms wide open, and I will always remember the impact I was able to have on one child's life through my service.

Thus inspired, I sought out more ways to make a difference and a classmate and I gathered hospital supplies, including 100 HIV test kits and lancets, and purchased gloves and alcohol pads. We helped test patients for HIV, a project that called on the knowledge and skills I acquired during my clinical rotations for the medical technology program. One of the most heartbreaking tasks I performed was informing an individual that he tested positive, but providing the peace of mind and prevention counseling to many men and women who tested negative gave me hope and left me with a great sense of accomplishment and a desire to do even more.

Wanting to learn more about the profession, I shadowed a PA and observed her as she diagnosed her patients' conditions and determined the course of treatment. Every consultation was an educational exchange where she learned more about the patient and their symptoms and educated them on preventative care, including proper nutrition and home-based exercise protocol. Her dedication to her patients only reinforced my decision to become a PA, as I was constantly reminded of the care my mother had received two years prior.

From my friend's encounter with a rock to coping with my mother's illness to my experiences in the field, I know that becoming a PA will allow me to lead a life of significance where I will directly impact lives and care for those in need. I look forward to taking the next step on this journey.

Essay 21 (812 words)

"One hundred twenty five, one hundred twenty six, one hundred twenty seven," I counted, as I waited for the second hand to reach one minute. The patient's pulse had increased at an alarming speed. As an emergency medical technician (EMT) I was the only certified health care professional in the gymnasium when the woman started experiencing chest pains and dizziness. She refused further medical attention and expressed the desire to drive home, but my instincts told me that she needed further medical attention. The gym owner left it to my discretion as to whether to call my squad for backup, and I knew the woman was trying to squelch her fear by refusing further medical treatment. I knew what I had to do.

I sat with the woman as I called the ambulance, and she began to relax as I explained how I could help her as an EMT-B. My psychology degree comes in handy as I address patients' emotional concerns, while my tactical emergency medical skills help me tend to patients' symptoms. On this occasion I presented the information to my fellow EMTs and relayed the status to the charge nurse when we arrived at the hospital via ambulance. I was glad to utilize my skill set and instincts to help this woman receive the care that she needed, and I long to impact many more people as a physician assistant (PA).

I experienced the life of a PA when I shadowed at Monmouth Medical Center. Despite their policy to only allow graduate students to shadow PAs, as an undergraduate student I knew I had to be persistent in order to attain my goals. My dedication paid off and I found myself shadowing physician assistants in the emergency department and volunteering in departments across the hospital. In my work with patients I witnessed the role of communication skills and bedside manner; my duties included serving as a liaison between patients and their health care team, relaying the patients' questions and concerns. Despite not providing physical care, I knew I had impacted the lives of patients and their families simply by giving them respect and attention. I am eager to marry my compassionate nature with the application of medical knowledge that PAs employ as they diagnose and treat patients.

Shadowing PAs in the ER and later at Seaview Orthopedics showed me the in-depth nature of their patient interactions. Not only do PAs order and interpret tests but they spend time with patients to thoroughly explain the results. Physician assistants also provide reassurance when a patient shows signs of unease; I remember a patient I encountered when shadowing Nadine, an orthopedic PA. He had suffered a complex injury that required a complex treatment plan, and Nadine took the initiative to draw a picture of his injury and what it would look like after treatment was completed, explaining the treatment and the recovery process. Despite her numerous responsibilities, Nadine never left a patient until they were satisfied with their treatment and all their questions were answered, and her approach taught me to show compassion to each individual rather than treating a patient like a chart number. Just as I immediately came to the aid of the woman in the gym, I will do the same with my future patients.

While shadowing various physician assistants I noted their relative autonomy and how when the PAs consulted with the physicians, their education and skills complimented the training of the physician. Observing this reminded me of the way a well-trained EMT crew works together seamlessly. Being aware of each other's abilities allows us to work fluidly while treating patients, and on emergency calls we anticipate what a fellow EMT might need or how our actions may impact them. My time as an EMT has prepared me to recognize the limits of my abilities and the importance of communicating with those with more medical authority.

I believe that physician assistants are so in tune with physicians because of the medical education credits they accumulate. The constant evolution of the medical field forces them to keep current with advances in medicine and technology. One PA explained to me that she had just earned credits toward her license by taking a quiz based on recent medical journals about developments across several areas of medicine. I am excited by the constant learning required, understanding that we must stay attuned to developments in the medical field. Through my determination, compassion, and experience I am confident that I will be an outstanding physician assistant, effective not only through my hands but through my heart as well. The gratification I gain from each encounter with the health care field has given me a taste of the incredible rewards I will receive during my career. I look forward to embarking on the next step of this journey to become a caring and healing physician assistant.

Essay 22 (522 words)

Giving up or getting discouraged by obstacles is simply not in my nature. The adversities I have faced have shaped my character and motivated me to keep moving forward at every turn. My decision to forge a new path as a physician assistant was not a change of career I took lightly, but once I set my mind to it, I never had a moment's hesitation.

It was the biggest decision of my life to leave a successful career in the music industry, the only career I knew and one to which I had devoted years of my life. My volunteer experience and years of work as an EMT in inner-city Atlanta left no doubt in my mind that this was the right decision. When you finally find something that you love and know is right, you will move mountains to get there. Moving those mountains requires patience and perseverance, and I have employed them both to get where I am. While my grades from over twenty years ago do not accurately represent my abilities, my more recent science coursework and efforts in my daily healthcare work better reflect my potential. I have always risen to the occasion, never shying away from difficult circumstances, and I feel these characteristics will benefit me as I embark on this next stage of my career.

My efforts over the past year and a half have moved me much closer to my ultimate goal of becoming a physician assistant. I have been working at a family practice owned by a husband and wife physician team with two PA's. It is a wonderful learning environment as the office handles everything from general medicine to urgent care. They are fantastic teachers who involve their team in the treatment of every patient so as to provide the best care possible. I am grateful for the opportunities and support they have given me, and I especially appreciate the opportunity to work as part of a true team. Whether in my career as a music manager, as an EMT or now as an MA, I have always thrived in a team environment. This is one of the many facets of the PA profession that appeal to me.

In addition to my demanding hours working at a busy family practice I continue to volunteer at the free clinic, one of my favorite places to be. It is inspiring to be a part of a team that provides such critical services to those who cannot afford care. It is also a challenging environment as approximately 90% of the patients speak Spanish and my Spanish is limited, but this experience has strengthened my commitment to my studies in Spanish.

While I wish I had found my passion for this path earlier in my life, I feel fortunate to have discovered it at all, recognizing that many people spend their entire lives searching for their true calling. Since beginning this quest towards a career as a PA I have gained substantially more knowledge, focus and wisdom—qualities that will serve me well and will be a tremendous assent on my journey towards becoming a PA.

Essay 23 (654 words)

I have known I was meant for a career in medicine ever since an incident in the summer of 1990. Some friends and I were playing a little rough when my friend Doris's toenail was accidentally ripped off. No adults were around, so despite the profuse amount of blood and Doris's hysterical crying, I knew we had to do something. My fear and nerves were no match for my intense desire to help Doris, so using a first aid kit from my parents' closet, I cleaned her wound and applied bandaging until her mom could get her to the doctor. Doris will probably always remember that day as traumatic, but for me, it was the day that I realized that practicing medicine was not just about taking vital signs and giving medication, but about giving patients the best care possible and peace of mind about their condition. I was hooked and knew that a career in medicine was my goal.

Upon my undergraduate graduation, I became an HIV/AIDS case manager in Camden, NJ where I worked closely with clients, families, social services, and medical professionals to coordinate services for people dealing with myriad life challenges. It was an invaluable experience that taught me to be empathetic and objective while focusing on the task at hand; I got up every morning ready to improve the health and wellbeing of my clients through care, compassion and respect. After serving as a case manager, I taught special needs students, not only providing daily instruction for them but tending to their basic medical needs as well. Because of my character and my passion for medicine, the school administration was confident in my ability to handle minor scrapes and bruises. Even parents of the most medically fragile students were comfortable with my first aid CPR training and my ability to react swiftly to emergencies.

While I gained valuable experience from serving as a HIV/AIDS case manager and from working with special needs students, the most significant aspect of both positions was the deep awareness I gained of the healthcare disparities between the affluent and the underprivileged. In communities where needs are the greatest, educational resources and quality of healthcare are the weakest. I knew I wanted to make a difference by pursuing a career supporting physicians serving urban communities.

I have both innate and acquired skills that will make me a successful physician assistant, recognizing that the requirements go far beyond empathy and awareness of societal injustices. In other professional roles, I have been deemed a highly competent leader, organized and assertive but never aggressive. I understand the competitiveness of the PA applicant pool, however, as a non-traditional student I bring maturity, preparation and confidence to my cohort. Since completing my bachelor's degree in psychology, I have completed upper-level science courses that have broadened my awareness and will help prepare me for a PA program. For example, in a recent genetics class, I researched the genetic disorder Osteogenesis Imperfecta and learned about the delicate process a healthcare team undertakes when a mother with this condition delivers a baby.

I am prepared for a rigorous course of study and for the practical experience that will lead me to a successful career as a physician assistant. I know what the job entails, as I have had the opportunity to observe physician assistants conducting physical exams, diagnosing and treating illnesses, ordering and reading tests, counseling patients on preventive care, writing prescriptions, and empowering patients. I have seen how physician assistants must act as independent thinkers and doers while also consulting closely with supervising physicians, and I understand the role that they play in a healthcare team. Moreover, my background as a case manager and public school teacher has prepared me to serve high-risk populations, which aligns with my goal of serving in urban communities. I look forward to giving as much back to the profession as I know it will give me.

Essay 24 (607 words)

After graduating from the University of Utah in 2003 with a degree in political science, I began my career as a lobbyist for public higher education in the great state of Utah. This was my dream job, or so I initially thought. I will always be grateful for the invaluable people skills I honed while lobbying on the Hill, not to mention the thicker skin I grew, but I was just not satisfied professionally. For several years following graduation I found myself pursuing numerous employment opportunities from being a dorm parent for troubled youth in rural New Hampshire to working as a legal assistant in a law office. I even thought about furthering my education in professional counseling or public administration and signed up for graduate classes. Even though each of these paths complimented my strengths and sparked my interest, none of them were quite the right fit. None evoked my true passion…until six years ago (enter choir: "Hallelujah! Hallelujah!"), when I discovered how rewarding and fulfilling being a physician assistant could be. I was hooked.

My metamorphosis began as a medical assistant in a large orthopedic practice where I worked with several physician assistants and their doctors. Though the doctors were impressive, it was the physician assistants who showed me the rewards of providing quality health care through patience, compassion and patient-centered approach. I was particularly inspired by the additional time the PAs spent with each patient, educating them on their ailment and explaining treatment options in layman's terms. This orthopedic group also treats the underserved migrant community in South Florida. I found this part of the practice especially rewarding, as I was able add medical terminology to my Spanish vocabulary while witnessing patient gratitude that was both humbling and motivating. Interacting with these patients made me long to be able to care for and treat them myself as a physician assistant.

Throughout my journey I have been fortunate to have exceptional mentors who encouraged me on my path towards becoming a physician assistant. I was advised to explore several areas of medicine, so in addition to orthopedics I worked and volunteered in dermatology, family medicine and urgent care. Even during the recession, when my hours were cut and jobs were scarce, I continued shadowing physician assistants and volunteered as a medical assistant on a regular basis. These very special practitioners instilled in me that the goal of every physician assistant is to ensure patient education, which in turn results in patient compliance and effective treatment. Thanks to them, my understanding of the role of a physician assistant is clearly defined as an extended care provider who delivers superior treatment. As an integral part of a health care team, I will assume the role of patient advocate and ensure that their needs are always met or exceeded.

I have spent the last six years preparing for this application process. Having found my perfect fit, I returned to school with a focus and drive like never before. Unlike my undergraduate coursework, where grades took a back seat to leadership and advocacy opportunities, I have dedicated myself to my academic preparation for the PA program and I am confident in my ability to perform in a demanding academic and clinical setting.

From my undergraduate activities in student development, leadership and advocacy, to writing and recording a hit song for ESPN, I am confident that I will add to the diversity and distinction of the 2013 entering class. I will fulfill the high standards of excellence commensurate with the physician assistant profession and will give back as much to the medical community as I know it will give me.

Essay 25 (495 words)

I am applying to the George Washington University Physician Assistant Program in order to advance my clinical knowledge and to gain the skills necessary to provide a higher level of patient care. Upon completion of the PA program, I plan to provide care to service-members wounded in combat and HIV/AIDS patients living in poverty, two under-served groups with which I am very familiar. I also plan to continue my research work as a Principal Investigator for clinical trials.

I earned a Bachelor of Science degree in Zoology and a Master of Science degree in Preventive Medicine from Ohio State University. The Preventive Medicine program focused on community and population health, biostatistics, and epidemiology. During college, I was employed as an Emergency Medical Technician (EMT) with the Ohio State University Emergency Medical Services and at the University Medical Center Emergency Department. For my master's thesis, I worked with the Ohio Department of Health, analyzing survey-question responses and the associated risk of HIV infection utilizing multiple-regression analyses.

After receiving my masters from Ohio State, I worked as a Clinical Data Analyst for a 350-bed hospital in Reno, Nevada, providing support to clinicians and hospital administrators in the identification of best practices and other quality improvement initiatives. I was promoted to Business Manager of Emergency, Trauma, and Surgical Services and was responsible for the financial health of each of these departments. I served in this position for two years.

For the last eleven years, I have worked in the pharmaceutical and medical device industries, managing clinical trials as a Clinical Research Associate. I have worked in many therapeutic areas: cardiovascular devices; infectious diseases including HIV and Hepatitis; endocrinology; pain management; auto-immune disorders like Crohn's Disease and Rheumatoid Arthritis; pediatrics for Type I Diabetes and vaccine clinical trials; etc.

I have been involved with community service beginning in my teens as a volunteer firefighter and EMT in my rural Ohio town. While living in Nevada, I was a volunteer technical search and rescue technician and EMT with the Washoe County (Reno) Sheriff's Office. Eighteen months ago, I enlisted in the US Army as a combat medic and currently serve with the US Army Reserve 75th Combat Support Hospital. I am a squad leader and responsible for organizing continuing education for the combat medics in my unit. I volunteer as a Community Outreach Representative with the Wounded Warrior Project. I am also training as an Honor Guard member, to serve at the funerals of service-members who have made the ultimate sacrifice.

All of my life experiences have lead me to this point and have created within me the passion and desire to provide my community and country with a higher level of care as a Physician Assistant. GW's commitment to community service and its diverse urban environment drew me to this program. As a graduate of GW's PA program, I will be able to serve my country and community by providing them with the level of care they truly need.

Essay 26 (852 words)

While volunteering at Second Wind, a riding stable for people with disabilities, I experienced profound joy at hearing an autistic child on horseback say her first word and seeing the ecstatic expression on a man's face when he realized that, even though he was paralyzed, he could still ride. As a physician assistant, I will have the opportunity and the privilege to influence people's lives positively every day.

My experiences at Second Wind and my love of science inspired me to major in medical technology. This healthcare-related field allowed me to study nearly every branch of science, and it seemed to be an ideal fit. I loved the coursework, and I especially enjoyed the focus on human pathology. My first job as a medical technologist was in a very small clinic. I enjoyed many aspects of my work, but I did not feel challenged and longed to utilize all my skills and training. I spent much of my time performing phlebotomy, and most of our samples were sent to a larger laboratory for testing. To prevent stagnation of my education and knowledge, I transferred to a larger lab.

I quickly realized that utilizing a more complex skill set was not enough for me to feel fulfilled. After a period of intensive introspection, I realized I need a career that includes direct interaction with patients. When the phlebotomists need assistance, I am eager to help them and to interact with patients. From providing therapy to autistic children to volunteering at Planned Parenthood, the highlights of my experiences have always been my direct interactions with patients. Although there is a patient connected with every lab sample, there is no face or personality for me to associate with it. I am an important member of the healthcare team, but I don't feel like a participant in individual patient care.

The best part of my first job was forming relationships with patients. As I prepared to draw blood from an elderly gentleman, I noticed that he had visited a doctor in another clinic that morning. When I informed him he could have had his blood drawn there instead of driving all the way across town, his response was, "I know that, but you won't screw it up." His words let me know how important it was for him to have someone he trusted draw his blood, and I felt honored to be that person. As a physician assistant, I will always be mindful that a patient's trust is an essential component of optimal healthcare.

I met another patient who came in regularly to have her Coumadin levels monitored. On her first visit, I asked her to be seated in the draw chair, and she burst into tears. She had recently undergone knee replacement surgery, was unable to tolerate her pain medication, and could not bend her knee enough to sit in a chair. The simple solution was to place a stool in front of the chair so she could keep her leg straight while sitting. On every visit thereafter, I made sure there was a stool ready for her, and on her final visit, she gave me a card to thank me for my patience and compassion. What I considered a simple act to provide comfort meant a great deal to this woman, and she confirmed that simple acts of caring make a big difference to a patient. My enthusiasm for my current work stems from the opportunity to employ my critical thinking and troubleshooting skills. My most important responsibility is to report accurate results for every test. Recently, I reviewed a patient's critically low calcium level, which had been normal just the previous day. It was obvious to me that this result could not be accurate and was not reported. These analytical skills and attention to detail will be invaluable when diagnosing a patient.

My participation in a Wilderness First Responder course through NOLS provided insights into comprehensive patient care. In this course, we learned to properly assess a patient, collect necessary history, provide treatment using few resources, and complete SOAP notes. To date, I have not utilized this knowledge in my field of clinical lab practice, but the classes made me aware of how much more I enjoy caring for the patient as a whole as opposed to performing strictly diagnostic testing.

My background as a medical technologist will give me an advantage as a PA. In addition to my familiarity with multitasking, I have a strong grasp of interpreting laboratory results, and I understand how these results are derived. I will know when to utilize a particular test method or identify potentially inaccurate results. Since most diagnoses utilize lab results in some form, my background will serve me well on a daily basis. As I reflect on the knowledge and skills gained from previous jobs, I feel especially well suited to a career as a physician assistant. I will be able to incorporate my critical thinking ability, my love of science, and my desire to care for individual patients as I pursue what I am convinced is the perfect career path for me.

Essay 27 (850 words)

As I regained consciousness, I wiped the blood from my eyes to see my mother standing over me. I was in the back seat of my best friend's rusted '67 Mustang that had collided with an ancient oak tree on a winding dirt road a mile from my home. My mother had been called to the accident site, not as the parent of her sixteen year-old injured son, but as an Emergency Medical Technician (EMT) with the volunteer service she and my father helped start just a few years prior. This accident would serve as the initial inspiration for a journey through many roles in healthcare, ultimately leading to my desire to become a PA.

I was rushed to the local Emergency Department (ED) with a ten-inch laceration to my scalp, and it was here that I had my first encounter with a physician assistant. He was a former Navy Corpsman like my father, and after the attending physician ruled out injury to my cervical spine the PA assumed responsibility for my care—an arduous and lengthy task of debridement and suturing. He showed concern for my pain and the emotions that were consuming my mother, periodically stopping to reassure us that although the injury appeared severe, with ample suturing and time it would heal without any permanent damage. As often happens with encounters during dramatic times, his calming nature and professionalism remains etched in my mind 25 years later.

Wanting to gain exposure to the medical field, during breaks from my freshman year of college I volunteered as a firefighter and EMT in my rural Ohio hometown and ended up working with the same PA who had cared for me two years prior. He always showed a keen interest in my education and experience as I transferred patient care over to the ED staff, asking me questions about the patient and taking time to answer my questions about diagnoses and treatments. His mentorship leads me to hope to do the same for future aspiring PAs.

During the remainder of my undergraduate and graduate years at Ohio State, I worked fulltime at the university Emergency Medical Services (EMS) and Medical Center ED as an EMT-Advanced. I thrived in the fast-paced environment of a Level I Trauma Center, fine-tuned my skills as an EMT, and came to know PAs and PA students rotating through the ED and Trauma Service. They were always enthusiastic and eager to document history and physicals, were skilled at performing procedures, and interacted in a meaningful way with all patients regardless of ailment or socioeconomic status. In addition to the experience gained, my graduate program in preventive medicine equipped me with the knowledge and skills to promote health through risk-reduction, disease identification and preventive medicine. I have employed these skills throughout my medical career and know that they will be key to my work as a physician assistant.

Having had meaningful clinical and educational experiences, I learned about the business of healthcare as business manager of Emergency, Trauma and Surgical Services for the largest hospital in Reno, Nevada where I balanced the compassion of caregiving with the business of healthcare and supplemented a physician shortage in a remote community with the skills and expertise of PAs. While I already held PAs in high regard, my respect for PAs only increased as I witnessed their dedication to providing uncompromised patient care in a high-pressure environment.

I spent the next eleven years managing clinical trials in the pharmaceutical and medical device industries, interacting with physicians, nurses, and PAs on a daily basis. During this time, I discovered that it was the PA in the medical practice who routinely consented the subjects for the clinical trial; the PA has the knowledge to answer the subjects' questions about the risks and benefits of the study medication as well as the patience and time to do so, providing an enormous service to the healthcare community in facilitating these trials.

After turning forty during the deadliest year of US military involvement in the Middle East, my focus turned to my lifelong goal of military service to my country. Refusing to live my life with any regret, and passing up officer commission, I enlisted in the US Army in order to serve as a combat medic. At the age of 41, I began basic training and the most rewarding and challenging eight months of my life. I am currently assigned to the 75th Combat Support Hospital where I work as part of a cohesive team of physicians, nurses, physician assistants and medics. The physician assistants in my unit have taken on a mentor the medics, inspiring us to preserve the lives of wounded soldiers on the battlefield. It has by far been the most powerful chapter of my life.

All of my experiences have culminated in a desire to advance my knowledge of the human condition and to gain the skills to aid my fellow man; these experiences have fueled my desire to become a physician assistant and I will give back as much to the profession as I know it will give me.

Essay 28 (649 words)

The last few years have been a time for me to reflect, review my career objectives, and plan for change. I want a medical career with a promising future and direct involvement with people. My future career must meet my need for continuing education, provide an opportunity for change, and utilize my past life experiences, training, and skills. The physician associate profession meets that criteria, and the viability of the physician assistant profession is without question. The creation of a national healthcare system that demands affordable healthcare will only intensify the need for PA's, and indicators suggest that this profession will grow throughout the next decade and beyond. I still have twenty to twenty-five working years ahead of me, and I want my next profession to be one that will offer both challenge and opportunity.

The role of a physician assistant goes beyond the treatment of symptoms and encompasses a deeper level of knowledge, compassion, and continuous learning. Most effective healthcare professionals have empathy for their patients, along with the required skills and expertise, but a physician assistant makes a greater contribution to society, and I am eager to fill that role. I look forward to making a contribution to my community and society.

For approximately fifteen years, I have been practicing as a chiropractic physician, and I have established a reputation for providing high-quality care to my patients. I have communicated and coordinated care with primary care phy-sicians and specialists in meeting patient needs. Most referrals to my practice come from other healthcare providers, and I attribute their confidence in me to my abilities as a team player and my understanding that a multidisciplinary approach is sometimes necessary. Having a family with small children made my decision to change careers a difficult one, but I feel it is best for my family and for our future. Years of adjusting patients, including the strenuous activity associated with the physical therapy and chiropractic techniques I utilize in my practice, are beginning to take a toll on my body. I enjoy what I do, but my job is physically hard on me, and I don't want to lose my passion for helping people because of it.

The other compelling reason for choosing the physician assistant career is that the profession has made tremendous advancements in the medical field, and it has worked to improve the future of the profession. I do not have those feelings about the chiropractic profession. We seem to have so many differing philosophies and agendas that, instead of growing stronger, we have alien-ated ourselves from one another. My goal is to participate in a profession that will continue to grow, become an integral part of our healthcare system, and develop the essential tools and resources necessary to best serve public health-care needs.

During my undergraduate years, I had to cope with my father's alcoholism and the effect it had on our family, and my academic performance suffered because of that. My grades in Chiropractic College, however, reflect my level of maturity and my commitment to succeed. Some of my extracurricular activ-ities, from elementary school through college, include my interest in music and my ability to play the Bouzouki, an ethnic Greek instrument. I formed a professional band that performed weekends at festivals, weddings, baptisms, and parties. To help finance my undergraduate education, I also owned and operated a hot dog concession stand during the summer months, and I worked at numerous jobs with a variety of people. These experiences greatly enhanced my communication and social skills.

An effective physician assistant collaborates with supervising physicians while maintaining independence and nurturing a good rapport with patients. My commitment to becoming a PA is unequivocal. During my career, I acquired the analytical, communication, and time management skills that will help me become a truly competent physician assistant, and I am confident that I will be an asset to the profession.

Essay 29 (758 words)

"Do it for the kids" is the motto of St. Jude Children's Research Hospital's Up 'til Dawn organization. This simple, yet powerful motto kept me motivated as I faced the daunting challenge of being a full-time student, full-time residence hall director, and committed leader of Illinois College's new organization, Up 'til Dawn. This organization raises funds and awareness for the children of St. Jude Children's Research Hospital. As the Executive Director of this organization, it was my responsibility to act as the liaison between Illinois College and St. Jude Children's Research Hospital. It was a collaborative effort which united faculty and staff with the students for one cause. Without the help and support of an outstanding team of committee chairs and committee members, we would not have been able to raise over $22,000 for the hospital. We truly "did it for the kids!"

I enrolled in Illinois College as a freshman during the fall of 2006. By the end of freshman year, I had decided to pursue a career as a physician assistant. My interest began when I was treated by a physician assistant who was a kind and knowledgeable healthcare professional. I wanted to have the ability to provide the highest quality patient care possible, while maintaining a calm and friendly atmosphere. Working as a physician assistant will allow me to work autonomously in providing patient care, while still giving me the opportunity to consult with a supervising physician on the more challenging and complex cases. I am pleased to know that as a physician assistant, countless opportunities are available as new interests arise. Regrettably, my first year at Illinois College was not spent giving adequate attention to my studies, and consequently, my grades suffered for that. I used this as a learning experience. I knew that if I was serious about being a physician assistant, I would need to buckle down to achieve my goal. While participating in many on campus groups, I was able to continuously increase my GPA through a combination of hard work, better time management and prioritizing my career goals. As I continued to challenge myself my senior year, I not only was able to take an 8 credit hour EMT-B course in addition to taking 19 credit hours at Illinois College for my undergraduate degree, but I was able to make the Dean's List both Fall and Spring semesters.

Just months after graduating from Illinois College and completing my undergraduate degree, I earned my EMT-B license. With a burning desire to work as a physician assistant, I continued to seek additional healthcare knowledge and experience. In an attempt to quench this yearning, I enrolled in an accelerated EMT-Paramedic course. Since July 2010, I have worked for LifeStar Ambulance in Jacksonville, IL gaining over 3,500 hours of direct patient care experience. Working in EMS has helped me gain a much better appreciation for the important roles that various team members play in providing quality patient care. Every day I go to work, I realize the impact we, the healthcare team, have on our patients' lives. There is a satisfaction felt deep inside when I make a difference in the lives of my patients and this fuels my passion to do more. With my experience working in EMS and working with other healthcare professionals, it is evident that physician assistants play an invaluable role in the healthcare system and I intend to become one of the best.

Through my experiences, I have successfully developed skills that will allow me to succeed as a physician assistant. Through my involvement in Up 'til Dawn and working as a hall director, I have gained valuable experience with groups of diverse individuals, as we establish common goals. Working as a paramedic has been beneficial and allowed me to expand on the skills I learned at Illinois College as I work within a healthcare team. Together, the care that we provide in collaboration with the many healthcare professionals at the hospital has proven how beneficial being a team player can be.

I have dedicated the past five years of my life preparing myself for the role as a physician assistant. My community service and educational pursuits have allowed me to mature, gain additional healthcare experience, and demonstrate my deep compassion for making a positive impact on the lives of others. I possess the dedication, desire, and determination needed to be successful in the physician assistant program. By successfully completing the physician assistant program, I will have the skills and knowledge required to provide outstanding care to my patients.

Essay 30 (505 words)

My desire to pursue a career in medicine as a physician's assistant is a product of my professional and personal background, my work ethic, and my desire to have a positive impact on the lives of others. For the past 15 years I have practiced chiropractic medicine, which has provided me with invaluable clinical experience in treating those ailments that respond to chiropractic modalities. Initially, it was the most rewarding endeavor of my life—the culmination of years of difficult schooling, clinical hours and hard work. However, with that same clinical experience and professional growth, I became increasingly frustrated with the limitations of chiropractic practice and felt that something was missing. I was searching for a common thread in medicine, a more comprehensive vantage point that would allow me to treat a broader spectrum of medical conditions so as to be of greater help to my patients. In my view, I was seeing just a piece of the puzzle, and not the entire solution.

Moreover, it was frustrating to have been educated in the medical model but to lack prescriptive authority. Ultimately, while I have enormous respect for chiropractic medicine as a means to an end, I became professionally unfulfilled and dissatisfied. It was this yearning to be a more complete healthcare practitioner that led me to pursue a career as a physician assistant.

Despite these philosophical concerns about my chosen profession, it was a recent life-altering experience that ultimately fueled my passion to make the change: my mother was diagnosed with lung cancer. While following the course of my mother's disease I had the opportunity to meet her doctors and interact with them on a professional level. Their dedication and tireless pursuit of the best possible treatment inspired me and re-ignited my own desire to pursue something more fulfilling. During this time, I became immersed in obtaining the best care possible for my mother, exhaustively researching the drug regimens and protocols best suited for her. Though it may sound a bit lofty, this personal mission further reinforced my belief that practicing medicine was my purpose in life.

In addition to my personal inspiration, I believe I have the right sets of experience to be successful in this field. Having practiced chiropractic medicine in inner city neighborhoods for the majority of my career, I have developed patience, understanding, and compassion from working with people of different cultures and ethnicities—traits that are essential when working as a physician's assistant.

I feel that my passion, dedication, clinical experience and maturity make me an excellent candidate for a program of your caliber. As an adult in my mid-forties and as a licensed chiropractic physician, I fully understand the commitment and stamina needed to meet the challenges of medicine and I possess the intellectual requirements and critical thinking skills needed to be an outstanding physician's assistant. I look forward to giving back as much as I know I will gain from the program and from the profession, and I respectfully thank you for your consideration of my candidacy.

Essay 31 (748 words)

In the trauma unit, I approached a new patient to obtain his consent for our Traumatic Brain Injury study. The patient wanted to go to the restroom, and I assisted him so he would not fall. Back in bed, he complained that he had not eaten lunch, so I found the duty nurse who told him he had already had his lunch and left the room. Becoming very upset, the patient started to cry and confided that his family, including his adult daughters and attorney brother, had abandoned him. Realizing his depression, I listened to him, encouraged him to be strong, and suggested he see a psychiatrist. After we talked for fifteen minutes, he felt better and appreciated my attention and respect. This experience greatly reinforced my desire to become a clinician and a director of patient care.

With my training and background as a clinician in China, it is now my dream to continue to direct patient care in the United States. I attended the Clinical Program at Xavier University Medical School where I did a fifteen-month U. S. clinical clerkship and sub-internship. During my training, I learned about the physician assistant profession and, for some of my rotations, I followed a PA when the physician was not available. The broad medical knowledge, accurate diagnosis, and sharp clinical skills of one PA impressed me enormously, and I admired his dedication to his patients and his satisfaction with his career. Later, when I worked as a medical assistant at a dermatology surgical center, I met another PA. After working with her, I gained an appreciation for the potential autonomy and opportunities for critical thinking that this career has to offer. As I learned more about the role of a PA, I realized this would be a better career goal for me than that of a physician. Not only can I take full advantage of my broad medical knowledge and clinical skills, but I can also fulfill a strong desire to continue my personal growth in the clinical field while having more time to fulfill my family responsibilities.

Having made that decision, I have devoted myself to preparing for PA school. I joined the AAPA, strived to obtain high GRE scores, took prerequisite courses or refreshers, and was able to shadow various specialty PAs at Parkland Hospital, St. Paul Hospital, and Children's Hospital. I learned that PAs have a unique role wherein they focus on an array of specialties under the supervision of a medical doctor but also work autonomously to assist physicians. Understanding the current challenges of the PA profession and the increasing demand for PAs, I am very passionate and excited about the opportunity to become a PA. Working as a volunteer at the West Side Clinic, a major volunteer community clinic providing limited primary care for the indigent and uninsured adults of Collin County, has provided me with another unique experience in this special clinical setting and reminds me of a homeless shelter in Atlanta where I once volunteered. These experiences will help me deal with similar situations in my future clinical practice.

The PA profession is very challenging, but I have a lot to offer, and my hands-on clinical experience in the United States will be a big advantage. As a clinical study coordinator for about three years, I often supervise junior study coordinators or mentor medical students with their research and heavy daily workload. This gives me the opportunity to use my excellent communication and interpersonal skills, provide efficient time management, and set priorities. I learned to be a team player and a team leader. Four years of teaching experience in medical school in China and in my U.S college has honed my excellent interpersonal skills. With more than three years of work experience in the information technology field, I am comfortable applying my computer skills within the medical field. In addition to my full-time job, and to improve my English as much as possible, I also participate in the Toastmasters Club. Interacting with my fellow members helps me to fine-tune my listening and speaking abilities, and these vital skills help me better understand and serve my patients.

My desire and commitment to becoming a physician assistant is so strong that I will not allow any obstacles to deter my progress. I intend to make the most of every opportunity to achieve this goal, and I look forward to bringing my strong motivation, reliability, interpersonal skills, and capacity for hard work to this program.

Essay 32 (620 words)

From my experience, positive outcomes are the most rewarding when achieved through hard work and perseverance. Through my trials of attempting to gain admission to physician assistant school, I have learned that preparation and time management skills are assets of achievement. In order to further my knowledge and better myself as a health care professional, I chose to re-take many of my science classes and continued to shadow physicians and physician assistants to learn more about the process that guides the decisions of those who operate in the health care field. I recently became a member of the Student American Academy of Physicians Assistants and the American Academy of Surgical Physician Assistants, associations that fuel my passion for the profession and through which I stay current in the field.

It is often through challenging circumstances that we are able to focus on what matters most to us. I recently suffered a tragic loss when both my parents passed away within three months of each other. Through their illnesses I became deeply involved in the care of both my parents, resulting in a renewed passion for the art of medicine. As the eldest of three children, I was called upon to make critical decisions related to my parents' care, a responsibility that made me acutely aware of the ethical trials that come with end of life decisions. With a heavy heart, I honored my mother's wishes to not be resuscitated while the rest of my family pushed desperately for a different route. My father suffered from a staph infection that caused his body to succumb to sepsis; despite my knowledge of the evils of sepsis, I honored my father's wishes of aggressive care in spite of the devastating ordeal he had just been through. When my father's condition deteriorated, I assisted the short-staffed team with CPR until more personnel could arrive. While obviously a heart wrenching time, I knew I had to maintain a positive and professional medical mindset.

Choosing my field of study was a simple decision, as I have been interested in medicine from a young age. While in high school I joined our local fire department and took EMT classes. As a rural department, our emergency services were the only medical services available for a thirty-mile radius, and this deep involvement sparked my dedication to helping others. As an adult, I was eager to pursue my paramedic licensure, and since completing the program I have maintained my EMT-B license and practiced emergency medicine.

I currently work at a Level 1 Trauma Center where I collaborate with physicians, physician assistants and other health care personnel on a daily basis. I have witnessed that the practice of health care is a team effort, and I have seen how communication and trust are key to solid team relationships. I have also gained experience as a technician in the surgical intensive care and burn intensive care units, roles that allowed me to examine labs, communicate with providers, and perform simple procedures like wound VAC care, assisting with skin grafts, and burn care.

I have the motivation, education, maturity and medical experience—including rehabilitation, wound care, emergency medicine, and critical care—to succeed in my pursuit of this degree and to become an outstanding physician assistant. I have the skills to assist and manage a team that will provide the best possible outcome for patients and their families, and I will apply a positive outlook to the intensive training that I will receive in the program. I look forward to taking the next step towards achieving my dream of becoming a physician assistant, bettering myself while embracing the education that will allow me to have a positive impact on the lives of others.

Essay 33 (838 words)

I am one of the lucky ones; the ones who know what they want to do with their lives. Today, more than ever, I know I want to become a physician assistant. The year 2009 had ups and downs that gave me insight about what I can do and gave me the wisdom to do it. My desire to become a physician assistant is inspired by my mom's battles with cancer, my dad's example as a physician in Ecuador, my personal experiences as an immigrant, and through my work serving the healthcare needs of underprivileged communities.

My mom was diagnosed with colon cancer in 2000 at the age of 72, her second time facing this devastating disease. Her disease affected me not only personally but professionally, and my experiences with her treatment inspired me to become a patient advocate. On one occasion, I went with my parents to my mother's doctor appointment and realized the many challenges and misunderstandings they faced. With only limited English skills, they didn't ask questions of the doctors or staff, just nodding and smiling to show respect. Another time, when my mom was receiving chemotherapy treatment, a lady sitting next to her asked for ice in Spanish but nobody understood her. I requested it for her and proceeded to translate a booklet of information for her. The gratitude she felt was only outweighed by my mother's pride watching me help this patient. Sadly, my mom lost her battle with cancer in 2002 but her healthcare experience, her courage and her words of inspiration made me realize that I wanted to pursue my dream of becoming a physician assistant.

The seed of working in medicine was planted long before my mother's illness, however, Growing up in Ecuador, I marveled at how caring and perceptive my father was with his patients and their families. I remember my dad showing me an amethyst and a quartz rock given to him as a symbol of appreciation and payment from a miner whose leg my dad had saved. I was so proud of my dad not only for saving the man's leg but for his openness to accepting these rocks as a form of payment. I began to picture myself following in his footsteps to help improve the lives of others.

After moving to the US, to gain more experience in the healthcare field I worked at a community health clinic in San Diego, where my language skills were invaluable. I remember assisting a Spanish speaking grandmother who suffered from diabetes. While conducting a health education session, I realized she had no idea what the physician had told her. Immediately, I called the doctor and interpreted for both. It is easy to take something as basic as understanding what someone else is telling you for granted, and I realized what a privilege it is to help someone understand her diagnosis and treatment. It also made me realize the deficiencies in a system where not every patient can understand what is happening to them, and further fueled my desire to advocate for patients as a PA.

Though I was accepted to a graduate PA program in 2009, a slippage in my grades prevented me from continuing. But over my two semesters there I learned a great deal, not only academically but about myself as well. I know what an intensive program looks and feels like; I struggled and overcame most of my academic challenges and my practical skills allowed me to demonstrate my strengths and interpersonal skills. I assisted with the H1N1 vaccination clinic where we served 2,000 residents of various ethnic backgrounds, and I performed physical examinations on the elderly at nursing homes. However, the program was not structured in a way that promoted student learning, and 75% of the class was placed on academic probation at the end of the second semester. The program lacked any support including tutors, and though I tried to receive help from instructors, their time was limited as they were working professionals. While preparing to reapply, I have learned new techniques to succeed in an academically intensive program. My passion for helping patients live healthier lives has not faltered, and I am committed now more than ever to becoming a physician assistant. I just need a second chance.

My experiences in life professionally and personally have prepared me for a career as a physician assistant. I believe that, like my dad, I have an innate ability to care for people and to help them with their medical care by relating to patients from other cultures and understanding their linguistic and cultural barriers. As a physician assistant I will have the tools to help underprivileged communities and to provide the best care for those in need. I am ready to live up to the challenge of becoming a devoted and successful PA. Roads take twists and turns but I am evermore sure of the path I have chosen. I look forward to giving back to the program as I know I will gain.

Essay 34 (523)

My first shift assignment at the hospital was transporting a patient back to his room. I introduced myself and saw that his left leg had been amputated, a complication of living with diabetes for over thirty-five years. He could not understand why I was willing to serve as a volunteer and he told me how the system had failed him. The center did not process his claims correctly, he explained, and their inefficiency made the process very difficult for him. Eventually, I had to turn my attention to my next assignment, but I promised him I would return. He looked doubtful, and when I did return later, he seemed stunned to see me again. He told me no one ever came back and the staff was constantly changing. As I continued our visits, we developed a friendly relationship. During our final visit, he wished me well and said I would be someone who could make a difference in the healthcare field. His confidence in me made me realize that a career in health care would be the best fit for me, and it strengthened my desire to play a significant role in patient care.

My volunteer efforts brought me into contact with many patients, and I learned to appreciate and value the relationship between patient and health-care provider. When volunteering at the Elgin Mental Health Center, I spent a great deal of time listening, counseling, and talking with patients, and these interactions were tremendously satisfying for me. Providing community-based counseling and support services that fostered hope, well-being, and self-esteem taught me a great deal. I learned the importance of empathy, support, and time spent listening to patients. Assisting patients with their recovery has enabled me to develop effective communication skills, and I have become proficient at teaching and sensitive in demonstrating compassion. It means a great deal to me when I hear patients say, "We can't wait for our next group discussion."

As an undergraduate, eager to provide a voice for those in need, I led various student groups and university departments in organizing programs that expose atrocities threatening the lives of people in many parts of the world. One of these programs was called, "Voices from Darfur," which promoted awareness of one of the most alarming humanitarian crises. I listened to the testimonies describing mental anguish and physical trauma and found it heart wrenching. As I listened to these stories, I became even more committed to the medical field and more passionate about helping others. As a physician assistant, I will work in public health at a significant level of medical intervention, and my heart will be as involved as my mind.

I enjoy direct contact with people in rapidly changing environments. I will welcome the opportunity to work directly with patients in serious need and enjoy using my analytical and time-management skills while drawing upon my community service experience. A career as a physician's assistant is one of the most rewarding in today's society, and I feel strongly that it is my true calling. I am confident I have a great deal to offer to those who need my help.

Essay 35 (828)

Exhausted, I urge myself to do just one more bicep curl. Next to me, a pair of elderly men are discussing test numbers and supplements. It is clear to me that one of them has just been diagnosed with prostate cancer. Immediately, I'm transported to the time I worked in research and the feeling of helplessness I experienced working in academia—this is why I need to be a physician assistant (PA). I could never return to research without being able to treat my patients.

Overcome, I realize that I need to be a PA. I must understand the details of how the body interacts with its environment and why. Moreover, I desire the capacity to address my patient's needs at a level that allows me to diagnose and prescribe treatment for them. At this point in my life, I have exhausted the idea of becoming a doctor, and do not want to spend the money or time earning the title, knowledge, and prestige associated with that career. I, Erin, need to be a PA because it would give me the opportunity to practice medicine and treat my patients in the shortest time possible—meeting my long-held desire to be a health care provider.

My journey has been long and lesson-filled, providing me with a strong foundation in humility, compassion, and empathy. I was born in the "Valley of Sickness" to a man crippled by multiple sclerosis, and a goal-oriented mother. Living in a rural area where people work at fast food restaurants and logging companies, we were surrounded by friends and family who lived on government checks. Accordingly, our loved ones suffered from poor mental and physical health. My family was not spared. My upbringing left me with an understanding of what it feels like to be helpless or "less than," which has been useful in helping me relate to my patients.

My life's mission is to serve those in need, and my thirst for science put me on the pre-medical track. In addition to taking a heavy course load, I worked as a nurse's aid and home health aide. My patients taught me about the value of life and to view the patient as a whole. These lessons helped me gain patient rapport, making me a better care provider. However, my work also taught me that I want to have a career with some level of autonomy, knowledge, and respect. Nursing did not seem to fit that mold, so I ruled it out as an option.

During the summer of my junior year of high school, I went to Ecuador to learn Spanish. Upon my return, I graduated a year early and attended Beloit College. While at Beloit, I studied off campus in Ashland, WI and again in Ecuador to become proficient in Spanish and to improve my understanding of minority populations (Ojibwa Indian and Quichua). These experiences were instructive, because they gave me a perspective on the way people around the world live. They also solidified my desire to work for people in need and to serve them. As a PA, I will recall these experiences and use them to identify with my patients.

Everything was on track, until I got sick during my junior year of college. The diagnosis stifled me, emotionally, not physically, for several years. I changed my focus in life, and decided to attend graduate school because I thought I was a different and lesser person. During my graduate education, I became more independent and confident in my abilities by conducting research in two areas: on methamphetamine consumption among women and epilepsy in Mongolia.

After earning my master's degree, I became a health educator for the health department. I supported the Clean Indoor Air Act by enforcing compliance, researching, creating, and promulgating literature. Also, my team and I cooperated to create and support minority and youth activist groups to reduce the impact of tobacco on the community. While my work was exciting and impactful, it did not "fulfill" me. So I decided to pursue research since it would get me a little closer to medicine.

Working as a research assistant allowed me to gain greater confidence in my work, improve my attention to detail, and increase my independent thinking ability. Most importantly, it allowed me to learn about the PA, MD, and NP profession first hand through discussion and shadowing. Those opportunities taught me that the PA profession is meant for me. From the moment I decided to become a PA, I have committed myself to the preparation for PA school by taking classes, joining PA academies, and reading current PA literature.

My abilities and experiences are uniquely suited for the PA profession. I have spent my life witnessing, working, and researching medicine. This has had a profound effect upon me, not only teaching me about medicine itself, but also imbuing me with a strong sense of empathy and compassion. My curiosity, intelligence and drive to treat the physical and emotional needs of my patients will make me an excellent PA.

Essay 36 (763)

A Ghanaian woman from the remote village of Kwame Danso flashed her hands twice and then held up four fingers indicating to the eye care team that she had lived with this blinded right eye for 24 years. The Unite for Sight team had evaluated this woman's condition earlier at their Charity Eye Clinic outpost and gave her five cedis needed to pay for transportation to the ophthalmologist's home for surgery. Originally, she had developed ptgeryium, which resulted in a corneal cyst and blindness. Through team effort, she received the much-needed surgery to remove the cyst. I'll never forget the woman's expression of joy with her restored vision. This woman had waited a long time as the eye condition did not hurt and she was not aware of Unite for Sight. During my stay in Ghana I worked with a team of local healthcare professionals providing care to patients living in extreme poverty. Every day, our eye clinic team traveled to remote villages on rugged dirt roads to provide eye assessments, care, and glasses to hundreds of patients. Seeing the grateful expressions of those we treated was an extremely moving experience. I felt fortunate to assist in surgeries that sometimes extended late into the night; witnessing the tireless and harmonious efforts of the local health professionals was both exhilarating and inspiring. Because the ophthalmologist had very little time with each patient, I felt a huge sense of responsibility, called upon as I was to dispense medication and provide patient education. I routinely relied on nonverbal communication as my understanding of Twi, their native language, was limited. My immersion into this quality team introduced me to the health care challenges facing developing countries, in particularly educating residents about availability of health care and treatment.

My interest in improving people's quality of life has deep roots. My father, an environmental engineer working at the EPA in Washington, D.C., focuses on maintaining safe drinking water. My mother, a neonatologist, brought me to the hospital many times as I was growing up, giving me early exposure to the health care community. I grew up with a clear view of the rewards, challenges, and sacrifices faced by health professionals.

My interest in patient care was augmented by my experience with Physician Assistants (PAs). In middle school, when I suffered an injury, I was profoundly impacted by my first interaction with a PA, who provided me with excellent emergency room care. After carefully examining my injury, she explained the need for an X-ray and the subsequent need to confer with the radiologist because the image was questionable. Thankfully, I did not have a fracture, but I was left with a very positive opinion of the PA's manner. During a previous emergency room visit for a foot injury, I did not see a PA, had automatic X-rays taken, and after a long wait, briefly spoke to a doctor. The contrast in careful, personable care with appropriate use of resources was immediately clear. More recently, a PA in a dermatology practice put me at ease with her excellent bedside manner. After conferring with the supervising dermatologist, she presented me with an easy-to-understand version of their conversation, making sure I understood the key details. I was so impressed with her that I will be shadowing her later this summer. I also plan to shadow other PAs in different specialties to enhance my understanding of the demands and rewards of my chosen career path.

Working as a full-time undergraduate research intern in the Advanced Imaging Group of the Queensland Brain Institute (QBI) significantly broadened my understanding of health issues, in particularly mental and neurological health challenges. QBI focuses on the diagnosis, treatment, and prevention of neurologic disorders. As the Advanced Imaging Group's only intern, I participated in several research projects using MRI analysis as related to the aging process, dementia, and familial epilepsy, on the published versions of which I'll be listed as a contributor. Realizing that medical care changes with time as new discoveries and treatments come to light, I understand the need to forever be a student, keeping up with new evidence upon which to base practice. With my full time research experience at QBI as a basis, I will review journal articles to provide current information to patients and insight to the hearth care team.

I believe that my background in neuroscience and research, when coupled with my demonstrated commitment to community service and my clear passion for patient care, makes me an excellent candidate for a PA program. I look forward to pursuing a career as a Physician Assistant.

Essay 37 (665 words)

I spent the first twelve years of my childhood living in Pakistan, where the standard of healthcare is marginal. When I was eleven years old, my grandfather suffered a heart attack and had to wait hours at the hospital before a health professional finally assessed his condition. He shared a room with five other patients, and although he pleaded for medical attention, the hospital staff did not respond. Even as a child, I knew that patients deserved better than this. My grandfather passed away later that day, and I will never forget my first exposure to the healthcare system or my resolve that someday I would change it.

My family and I moved to the United States soon after my grandfather's death. As I progressed through elementary and high school, I was confused about which direction to take in the medical field, and I struggled with my options of becoming a doctor, nurse, or physical therapist. None of these career paths seemed right for me, but I knew I wanted to work as part of a team while having the responsibility and autonomy to make my own decisions in patient care.

In 2005, a devastating 7.6 magnitude earthquake hit Pakistan, and the Islamic Relief Foundation requested the help of volunteers. Even though I was enrolled as a full-time college student, I decided to volunteer for ten days in the relief effort. I saw this as an opportunity help others as well as develop my skills as a member of a healthcare team. In the process, I was deeply moved by the devastation caused by the earthquake and its impact on infants, children, adults, and elderly people of all backgrounds and socioeconomic conditions.

I continued my college education after returning from Pakistan, but my mother was diagnosed with a malignant blood disorder in 2007, and my sense of helplessness was overwhelming. During her treatment process, a physician assistant, Aamir Khan, was assigned to her medical team, and I experienced my first contact with this profession. Mr. Kahn and I developed a professional and educational mentorship, and he advised me to enhance my knowledge and skills and begin my healthcare career by working as a nurse technician at a local clinic. While shadowing Mr. Khan in a clinical setting, I learned more about the role of a physician assistant, and this experience confirmed my decision that this would be my future career.

Over the next two years, I continued working as a nurses' aid at the local clinic, working closely with patients, taking vital signs, and collecting short medical histories. We also volunteered and organized free screenings and seminars to educate those within the community and assisted with seminars advocating primary prevention measures such as exercising and smoking cessation. These efforts helped me grow as a healthcare provider and further enhanced my skills and professionalism.

Last year, I applied to several physician assistant programs but was not accepted. I realized I was not up to par with other applicants, and knew I had to strengthen my candidacy. I contacted faculty from each university that had invited me for an interview and asked for their feedback. Acting on their advice,

I returned to school in the summer to improve my academic record. I repeated one of my courses and improved my grade from a B to an A. I also worked full time as a certified personal trainer, which gave me even more exposure to direct patient care. My colleagues and I established a volunteer based community initiative to teach local children the importance of physical exercise and proper nutrition, and I registered as an affiliate member of the American Academy of Physician Assistants. I am proud to have taken advantage of this opportunity to improve myself, both professionally and personally. When my grandfather died, I had a dream of becoming a healthcare provider and making a difference in the lives of others, and I am determined to overcome any future challenges no matter what is required of me.

Essay 38 (1151 words)

I have desired to be a physician assistant literally since the time I discovered what a PA is. Two things set in motion my dream of becoming a PA: First I have had a desire since childhood to help people. The examples shown by both my father and grandfather as ministers were ever present influences on the desperate need of the human heart for healing, as well as the gratification that serving them and helping in the healing process can bring. My heart was stirred to help people.-I went on various missions trip with my church to a native American reservation and to Mexico and I witnessed the health needs of the people there, both physically and mentally. The secondary source of inspiration came due to meeting with and being treated by a PA at my doctor's office. Her personable and kind manner set me at ease, and she was truly professional in her work. The initial encounter with that PA caused me to begin to investigate what was involved with becoming a physician's assistant. I shadowed two of the PA's that worked at my doctor's office, as well as a urologist who allowed me to assist in a supervised capacity in several surgeries. Even being given a small taste of the experience of assisting filled me with excitement and passion. The more I researched the role, the more intrigued and challenged I became, to the point of it becoming the professional dream of my life.

The process of learning has always been, and will doubtless continue to be a source of great enjoyment for me. Because good grades had always come easily to me, I misjudged my natural academic strengths when it came to certain college level classes. The mistakes I made related to overloading myself with class and work hours' cost me dearly. While I did well as a rule, my math and chemistry class struggles caused me to put my dream on hold and I learned the hard way that in order to succeed academically, I can never make the assumption that a class is easy.

My study focus and efforts required a long hard look, as well as personal scrutiny. After re-evaluating my time management and study techniques, I graduated with my master's degree in counseling psychology. Upon completion of my degree, I was required to pass a difficult exam in order to obtain licensure as a professional counselor, as well as complete 3000 hours of supervised experience. Since that time, I have been employed by Kingwood Pines Hospital for 3 years. While I enjoy interaction with people in their mental and emotional health needs, my dream of becoming a PA never died. In place of the discouragement I had toward becoming a PA, I began to see a strength of combining my ability as a counselor and that of being a PA as one final challenge I was ready to conquer.

With the encouragement of my family and professional colleagues, I felt encouraged to renew my dream of becoming a PA. Equally important to me was proving to myself as well any school that I would attend that I can make good grades and successfully master the math and chemistry courses that stumped me before. Rather than taking short summer courses, as I had before, I carefully and methodically planned my path to success. This meant returning to college and taking over not only the classes with undesirable grades, but also those in which I wanted to have a current and refreshed knowledge. Likewise, the chemistry classes were postponed until after I had spent a semester working individually with a tutor to ensure that I had a firm foundation and comprehension of the subject. Not only have I passed these classes but my grades were superior enough that the dean extended an invitation to join the honors program. My commitment is for this momentum to continue to spur me on to success throughout all remaining courses.

While nobody likes making mistakes or periods of uncertainty, I believe that my experiences have endowed me with more compassion and understanding than I could have had without them. In dealing with patients, I recognize that many of their health problems will likewise result from poor personal choices, but they are in no less need of my compassion. The listening skills and empathy I have cultivated in my practice as a counselor will only serve to embellish the care I hope to provide. Certainly in my dealings with people, I have worked with various personalities many would initially view as challenging or off-putting, but my experience has sharpened my clinical judgment and increased my confidence and assertiveness. My approach will be one of humility, and born of a true appreciation to serve and care for others.

In keeping with this background, I feel that Baylor is the ideal choice for pursuing my education as a PA. After attending an information session, I was struck by the program director's words that he views the program as a finishing school of sorts, where the students are fine polished until they can shine. My desire is to reach my fullest potential, and this statement revealed to me an attitude that the faculty shares in that desire. While at a graduate level, the burden of academic success ultimately rests on my shoulders, it is encouraging to know that instructors will support and motivate me as well.

As a Texas resident, Baylor's name is a familiar one to me. Before learning the formal history of either the school, or the medical facilities, I was introduced to Baylor as a little girl when my grandfather underwent heart surgery in one of its Dallas-based hospitals. In college, I visited a friend at the Waco campus, and the animal lover in me was impressed and excited that they kept bears onsite! Also, as recently as last year, a dear friend of mine faced a life-threatening situation, and it was at another Baylor facility that she received the care she needed to survive.

On an academic level, Baylor impresses me as unparalleled. The ranking in U.S. News and World Report as the nation's ninth leading PA program speaks for itself of the fine education and training its graduates receive. The rigors of a career as a PA demand a comprehensive and meticulous preparation period, and I believe that Baylor will best equip me to meet those demands.

I feel I can flourish in the role of a PA, and if I am fortunate enough to attend Baylor's program, I will do so with the finest of education to support me. My determination has driven me to excel, my previous experiences have taught me that hard work has become my friend, and mediocrity my sworn enemy. The achievement of this goal will propel me to higher personal and professional heights, and truly be the realization of a lifelong dream.

Essay 39 (693 words)

It was a sunny and humid day in the shanty town of Caracas, Venezuela. My surgical gown was damp and my mask stuck to my balmy face. Kids' laughter filled our ears and eased my nerves as they chased each other, barefoot, around the rocky terrain outside of our medical tent. It was the first time I had aided a delivery, let alone one with minimal medical supplies and hours away from a hospital. Ofelia, a young pregnant mother, gripped my hand as I counted down from ten. One last push, and the baby appeared. I helped the doctor drain fluid from his sinuses with a bulb syringe and Ofelia's eyes filled with tears as she heard her son's long awaited first cries. I can still hear her voice as she cried out "Gracias a Dios por ustedes!" (Thank God for you all!). It was in that moment, when I carried Gabriel's fragile body to his mother and sprawled him over her chest, that I realized how delicate life is. I remember gazing at the world around me and realizing that beyond language barriers, socioeconomic status, and cultural differences, we are all the same. Experiencing such profound satisfaction in helping those without the medical care they rightfully deserve inspired me to return with the appropriate medical training to further help those in need.

The miracle of medicine and the human body has never failed to astonish me. From a young age, I shadowed my father on his hospital rounds and imagined I was a health care provider as I scribbled in his patients' charts. I still have my life size anatomy and physiology coloring book that I would use to diagnose my imaginary patients. Although I admired my father's ability to manage his relentless health care service while providing his utmost support to his family, I dreamed of a profession that required less business management and focused more on patient care. Towards the end of my sophomore year of college, my father unexpectedly suffered from a stroke. My invincible hero now lay on a hospital bed, plugged into machines. I suddenly and painfully understood what it was like to be on the other side of the curtain. One night, as I sat bedside by my father, a physician assistant walked in to check on him. She asked a few questions and proceeded to check his heartbeat. She must have felt my worry since she looked at me and warmly asked, "Want to listen?" I had seen many physician assistants before that night, but this my first interaction with one. Meeting her that night, and witnessing the expertise and the compassion that she brought to her patients and their families, fueled my desire to become a PA.

I began to research the PA profession and developed relationships with a few who allowed me to shadow in different health care settings, such as nursing homes, hospitals, and clinics. Each impressed me with intelligence and empathy, always composed, yet able to work efficiently under pressure - qualities that I admire and patient care that I commend. They worked as a healthcare team, as opposed to the more independent healthcare I had witnessed most of my life. They comforted patients and thoroughly explained circumstances, as opposed to speaking in ambiguous medial terms. I continued working as a medical assistant at a healthcare clinic but lightened my load in my senior year, which I felt improved my academic performance. I found great reward in volunteering at the free Huda clinic in the underserved Detroit area. I worked mainly as a Spanish and Arabic translator, which inspired my medical aide trip to Caracas, Venezuela last summer. It was after my experience in South America that I felt a true calling to help those in particular who are less economically advantaged.

My father once told me, "You can be anything you want, as long as you put your mind to it." I am confident that I can and will achieve my goal of becoming an exceptional physician assistant. I look forward to the day when I hold the stethoscope up to a patient's ear and ask, "Want to listen?"

Essay 40 (539 words)

I have encountered many people and experiences in my life, but few have impressed upon me the deep desire and zeal to attend PA school like dancing with the Minnesota Ballet and teaching with Teach For America. These two very different yet definitive experiences changed and prepared me in profound ways.

While dancing for the Minnesota Ballet I was chosen to be the lead role in the Nutcracker. It was opening night and as I walked onto the stage feeling the warm lights and hearing the faint beginnings of the orchestra playing the first overture my mind turned off and the excitement and passion to perform took over. It wasn't until the standing ovation, I reflected on all of the hard work and rehearsals that encompassed this profound and exciting experience. The Nutcracker performance was a moment I will never forget. In retrospect, I see the tremendous lessons I learned at an early age about passion and the incredible amount of hard work, discipline, teamwork, and enthusiasm it involved. Ballet was the first glimpse into my eventual pursuit into the PA profession.

Long after I set my ballet slippers aside I felt the familiar deep-rooted passion when I worked in a low-income middle school. I wrote the following in my journal half way through my Teach For America experience: "I am now two days over half way and realize the changes in who I am and in who my students are becoming. I visualize my student's faces, especially those moments that seem to be ingrained in my brain like a snapshot photograph. I see the face of one student as he admitted to me his involvement in gangs, the proud face of another student as he saw his 98% test score and even took it to the bathroom so no one could steal it. I see the tears in still another student's eyes because he's not at home caring for his mother, and the tears streaming down a mother's eyes as she pleads for any advice on how to raise her child." These are merely just a few of the moments that I realize have changed who I am. My Teach For America experience was much more profound than what I could've ever imagined. Each difficulty I persevered through I see myself as a more dedicated, passionate, and enthusiastic individual willing to serve despite the possibility of facing demanding circumstances. More so, I learned a new perspective, creativity, and desire to learn science and medicine through teaching others. I relished educating others about medicine and science yet I felt a strong desire to pursue a career that extended even further beyond the classroom.

I've learned the significance of working hard and persevering through tough circumstances for something I deeply desire. I have been strengthened and challenged through these experiences in what it means to not only be dedicated but also passionate. Subsequently, I discovered the PA profession encompasses the very things I had desired from my previous experiences. In my pursuit to attend PA school I anticipate the hard work, the challenge, and to face difficulties. I am confident I am fully prepared through what I've learned to carry each lesson forward with a fervor for medicine and a dedicated heart to serve.

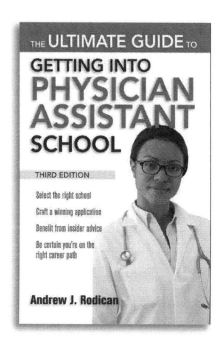

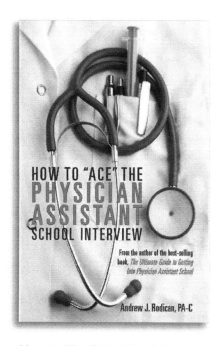

The Ultimate Guide to Getting into Physician Assistant School is a step-by-step blueprint for succeeding at every stage of the PA application process. Clear and candid, this book provides insights, information, and advice you won't find anyplace else— but may well make the difference between the acceptance or rejection of your application.

How to "Ace" the Physician Assistant School Interview will give you the competitive edge at the physician assistant school interview with step-by-step instructions that covers the entire PA school interview process. It will boost your confidence, arm you with knowledge, and you'll know exactly what to expect.

Made in the USA
Middletown, DE
06 June 2016